# Bronchopulmonary Dysplasia
## Strategies for Total Patient Care

**Edited by:**
*Carolyn Houska Lund, RN, MS*
*Children's Hospital*
*Oakland, California*

***Neonatal Network®***
191 Lynch Creek Way, Suite 101
Petaluma, CA 94954-2313
(707) 762-2646

**Book design and composition by:**
**First Impressions**
Marsha Godfrey

ISBN: 0-9622975-2-6

# TABLE OF CONTENTS

## Contributing Authors:

Susan Arndt Park, RN, BSN
*Harborview General Hospital*
*Seattle, Washington*

Donna Carson, MSW, MED
*Emory Regional Perinatal Center*
*Atlanta, Georgia*

Sharon Boatright Collier, RD
*Children's Hospital*
*Boston, Massachusetts*

Linda Corcoran, RN
*Children's Hospital of Philadelphia*
*Philadelphia, Pennsylvania*

David J. Durand, MD, FAAP
*Children's Hospital*
*Oakland, California*

Linda S. Franck, RN, MS
*Children's Hospital*
*Oakland, California*

Lily C. Kao, MD, FAAP
*Children's Hospital*
*Oakland, California*

Carolyn Houska Lund, RN, MS
*Children's Hospital*
*Oakland, California*

Bruce Nickerson, MD
*Children's Hospital*
*Oakland, California*

Rosalyn Feller Scherf, RNC
*Northshore Medical Center Hospital*
*Miami, Florida*

Kathleen A. VandenBerg, MA
*Children's Hospital*
*Oakland, California*

Jean Zander, RN, MSN
*James Witcomb Riley Hospital for Children*
*Indianapolis, Indiana*

# Introduction

The appearance of chronic pulmonary disease as a sequelae of acute neonatal lung injury combined with mechanical ventilation has provided health professionals in the neonatal intensive care nursery with a challenge that few had anticipated. Neonatal intensive care was initiated as an acute care specialty concerned with neonates born prematurely or with serious disease or malformations. The heroic efforts directed toward these neonates in the early days of their existence were the focus of research and education for health providers; the literature abounds with information on resuscitation, stabilization and other aspects of acute management for critically ill neonates. Care for infants with chronic disease, in this case bronchopulmonary dysplasia or BPD, calls for different approaches than those practiced with acute neonatal illnesses.

BPD represents a wide spectrum of illness. This includes the infant recovering from respiratory distress syndrome with a slightly abnormal chest x-ray and borderline pulmonary function tests who breathes room air and nipples well, the infant who requires several months of oxygen therapy via nasal cannula to support growth and prevent subtle respiratory compromise, the infant who is ventilator dependent for six months or longer, and the infant whose course lies somewhere in between these examples. There is growing interest in how to prevent or minimize the development of BPD in neonates, as well as how to best care for infants who are developing and recovering from BPD in the NICU. It is to this latter topic that we devote this monograph.

The authors of these chapters represent a variety of disciplines devoted to clinical care for infants with BPD. We begin with a discussion of the pathogenesis of BPD and an overview of current therapies. Respiratory management is then explored, as well as the numerous complications seen as a result of lung damage or long term hospitalization. Pharmacologic therapies are presented along with a discussion on pulmonary mechanics in BPD since these are becoming more available and are extremely useful to determine the efficacy of various medication regimes.

Nutrition plays a key role in the recovery from BPD, and is detailed from early parenteral nutrition approaches to the introduction of oral feedings. Due to the prolonged hospitalization and limitations of compromised lung function on comfort and development, an extensive chapter discusses the issues of behavior and agitation in the care of infants with BPD. The impact of chronic disease and lengthy separation of infants from their families is described in interviews with two families about their experiences. The final two chapters look at the process involved in discharge planning for more complex infants with BPD who may require special equipment, pulmonary follow-up for months to years, or even home ventilation. The appendix includes checklists for elements of discharge, as well as nursing care plans for the hospitalized infant with BPD.

For the future, our hope lies in the prevention of prematurity, in early therapies that minimize the damage caused by mechanical ventilation such as surfactant replacement, high frequency ventilation and extracorporeal membrane oxygenation, and in strategies that promote better healing for injured lung tissue such as vitamin A and antioxidant agents like the enzyme superoxide dismutase. Our hope for the present is that we will devise strategies to help infants and their families recover from BPD in ways that minimize the negative effects of longer hospitalizations and separation from normal family life.

## Dedication

*To my father, Charles Houska, who taught me about hope.*

CHAPTER 1

# An Overview of Bronchopulmonary Dysplasia: Pathogenesis and Current Therapy

*Bruce Nickerson, MD*
*Children's Hospital*
*Oakland, California*

Bronchopulmonary dysplasia (BPD) is the chronic lung disease that some infants develop after an acute episode of respiratory failure. Northway, Rosan, and Porter coined the term in 1967 to describe the roentgenographic changes seen in the lungs of premature infants who survived severe hyaline membrane disease.[1] A similar clinical syndrome may also occur after respiratory failure due to other causes such as bacterial or viral pneumonitis, meconium aspiration, or chronic cardiac failure.

Bronchopulmonary dysplasia is now defined as the chronic pulmonary condition of infants who have experienced respiratory failure, remain oxygen dependent for at least 30 days, and have chronic pulmonary pathology with chest x-rays that reveal areas of hyperinflation and areas of atelectasis. There is a wide spectrum of illness, from infants who have mild symptoms to those who remain ventilator dependent for many months.[2]

Bronchopulmonary dysplasia is reported in 15–38 percent of infants weighing less than 1,500 gm who require mechanical ventilation for hyaline membrane disease. Advances in neonatal intensive care have resulted in a changing pattern and incidence of BPD: Improvements in techniques for

**TABLE 1 ■ Etiologic Factors Associated with Bronchopulmonary Dysplasia**

| | |
|---|---|
| ***Prematurity*** | ***Infections*** |
| ***Hyaline membrane disease*** | Bacterial pneumonia |
| ***Surfactant deficiency*** | Viral pneumonia |
| ***Oxygen toxicity*** | ***Aspiration*** |
| ***Barotrauma*** | Meconium |
| Pneumothorax | Blood |
| Interstitial emphysema | Gastric acid |
| ***Cardiac failure*** | ***Genetic*** |
| Patent ductus arteriosus | Predisposition to reactive airways |
| Other congenital heart disease | |
| Fluid overload | |

mechanical ventilation that have prevented the disease in some infants have also allowed more of the tiniest and sickest infants, who are at high risk for BPD, to survive. This chapter outlines the etiology, clinical course, complications, and treatment of BPD.

## Etiology

Bronchopulmonary dysplasia has a multifactorial etiology (Table 1) that is mediated by the inflammatory reaction. Inflammation may be brought on by pulmonary oxygen toxicity, mechanical trauma from the ventilator, or the underlying disease process itself. Factors such as infection, pulmonary edema due to fluid overload or cardiac disease, and familial predisposition to reactive airways may also play a role.

### Oxygen Toxicity

When Joseph Priestly discovered oxygen, he observed that rats placed in 100 percent oxygen die from respiratory disease within two days. In these animal models of acute oxygen toxicity, the lungs are edematous with areas of hemorrhage. At a fraction of inspired oxygen ($FiO_2$) between 50 and 80 percent, pathological changes of oxygen toxicity take longer to develop; at an $FiO_2$ below 40 percent, the changes of oxygen toxicity are difficult to demonstrate.

The mechanism of oxygen toxicity appears to be through oxidant damage to cells which attracts polymorphonuclear leukocytes to the lungs and causes them to release inflammatory mediators, which further oxidize cell membranes and cause even more inflammatory changes (Figure 1). Pulmonary defenses against oxidant damage include glutathione, superoxide dismutase, catalase, vitamin E, and some lipids. Oxygen damage causes progressive breakdown of

**FIGURE 1 ■ The Mechanism of Oxygen Toxicity**

Oxygen
↓
Oxidant damage to cells
↓
Release of chemotactic factors
↓
Migration of inflammatory cells to the lungs
↓
Release of mediators or inflammation
↓
Fibrosis

the endothelial barrier with leakage of protein, fluid, and eventually frank hemorrhage into the interstitial spaces and alveolae.[3–6]

### Barotrauma

Infants and animals who are chronically ventilated, particularly at higher pressures, develop inflammatory changes and leakage of fluid into the interstitial spaces. Several investigators found BPD to be more prevalent among infants ventilated with greater than 35 cm of water pressure; when the approach to ventilation was changed to consistently use lower peak inspiratory pressures the incidence of BPD was less prevalent.[7,8] Other investigators report a relationship between high airway pressure, pneumothorax, and pneumomediastinum and the later development of BPD, suggesting that excessive airway pressure as the common factor.[9–12]

Because there is a trade-off between airway pressure and oxygen requirements, clinicians must choose between increasing either pressure or inspired oxygen concentrations to obtain adequate gas exchange. Infants already suffering from BPD may have such severe lung disease with decreased compliance and poor gas exchange that they require high airway pressures and oxygen concentrations to survive. There may be some mechanical and biochemical adaptations that allow these infants to survive chronic exposure to such conditions. For example, infants with chronic BPD rarely suffer from pneumothoraces. The recent development of techniques for high-frequency ventilation for RDS may allow for oxygen delivery at lower mean airway pressures. There is hope that this experimental therapy will increase survival with decreased barotrauma when adequate experience with its use has been accumulated.[13–15]

### Pulmonary Edema

Bronchopulmonary dysplasia has been common among infants who experi-

**TABLE 2 ■ Stages of Bronchopulmonary Dysplasia and Their Complications and Treatments**

| STAGE | COMPLICATIONS | TREATMENTS |
|---|---|---|
| ***Stage I*** | | |
| Severe hyaline membrane disease | Respiratory failure | Oxygen, continuous positive airway pressure, ventilation |
| | Bacterial infection | Antibiotics |
| | Air leaks | Chest tubes |
| | Intraventricular hemorrhage | |
| ***Stage II*** | | |
| Severe lung disease | Patent ductus arteriosus | Surgery, indomethacin |
| | Pulmonary edema | Diuretics |
| | | Fluid restriction |
| ***Stage III*** | | |
| Transition to chronic lung disease | Failure to wean from ventilator | Oxygen |
| | Carbon dioxide retention | Bronchodilators |
| | Interstitial pulmonary edema | Diuretics |
| ***Stage IV*** | | |
| Chronic lung disease | Tracheal stenosis | |
| | Cor pulmonale | Oxygen, diuretics |
| | Gastroesophageal reflux | Metoclopramide, surgery |
| | Growth failure | Increased calories |
| | Interstitial pulmonary edema | Diuretics |

ence congestive heart failure from a patent ductus arteriosus requiring surgical ligation.[16] It is unclear whether pulmonary edema itself or the increased requirements for oxygen and airway pressure account for this association. More aggressive management of patent ductus arteriosus with improved echocardiographic diagnosis, medical treatment with indomethacin, and early surgical ligation if medical therapies fail have decreased but not eliminated the importance of this factor.

One study found that infants who later developed BPD had received more fluid in the first days of life than infants who did not develop BPD.[17] This finding has led neonatologists to decrease fluid intake in infants with respiratory disease and to carefully monitor fluid administration. The thin skin and the large surface area relative to the mass in infants weighing less than 1,000 gm lead to large insensible losses, so fluid balance is precarious.

### Prematurity

Premature delivery and spontaneous respiration may also affect pulmonary development. Subtle decreases in small airway functions were demonstrated in 6 to10 year old children who had been premature infants without hyaline membrane disease.[18] Thus, breathing by underdeveloped lungs may affect their subsequent development.

### Inflammatory Damage

Adults and older children experiencing insults to the lungs, such as pneumonia or shock lung requiring high inspiratory pressures, may develop chronic lung disease similar to BPD. Therefore, inflammatory processes themselves, without prematurity, may predispose the small infant to develop BPD.[19-26]

### Genetic Predisposition

Genetic factors may also be important. Male infants, infants with inherently small airways, or those with a genetic predisposition to reactive airways appear to be more susceptible to lung insults.[27]

## Clinical Course

We have adapted Northway's radiographic classification to reflect the clinical course of BPD. Table 2 summarizes some of the common complications and treatments of BPD as they arise in each of these stages.

### Stage I: Hyaline Membrane Disease

Bronchopulmonary dysplasia usually begins as severe hyaline membrane disease in tiny premature infants, most often in those who are 12–16 weeks premature. Initially, their status is characterized by severe hypoxemia despite oxygen therapy, diffuse microatelectasis, and decreased compliance of the lungs. Treatment with mechanical ventilation may be complicated by pneumothorax, and these infants may also suffer from birth asphyxia or intraventricular hemorrhage.

### Stage II: Severe Lung Disease

Instead of the usual course of hyaline membrane disease with diuresis and pulmonary improvement on the third or fourth day, infants who develop BPD require continuing oxygen therapy and show a "white-out" of the lungs on roentgenograms. This stage is associated with the development of congestive heart failure, usually due to a patent ductus arteriosus. Better recognition of patent ductus arteriosus with echocardiography and medical therapy with diuretics and indomethacin have decreased the frequency of this complication.[28] Infants may develop BPD without ever showing the radiographic changes that characterize this stage.

### Stage III: Transition to Chronic Lung Disease

This transitional stage occurs at some point during the first month of life. These infants improve somewhat but still require oxygen and may fail to wean from mechanical ventilation. Chest x-ray films show a diffuse bubbly appearance with alternating areas of overdistension and atelectasis. The infant may have episodic wheezing and cyanosis. Carbon dioxide levels often rise despite mechanical ventilation. Common complications include feeding intolerance, aspiration, and sepsis. The current therapy frequently includes diuretics and bronchodilators.[29,30]

### Stage IV: Chronic Lung Disease

At one month of age, infants with BPD are easily distinguishable from those who have recovered. Infants with BPD require supplemental oxygen and/or mechanical ventilation; many also receive regular doses of diuretics and bronchodilators. Radiographs often show hyperinflation with areas of atelectasis and overdistension. If lower pressures are used, the degree of hyperinflation can often be decreased. By this time, the tracheal aspirate contains inflammatory cells.[31,32] Figures 2 through 5 illustrate the progression of BPD in the radiographs of a single infant on the first, ninth, twentieth, and seventy fifth days of life.

A frequent problem is very labile pulmonary function with episodes of severe cyanosis, wheezing, and decreased compliance. The exact pathophysiology of this phenomenon is still not well studied.

Infants with BPD commonly have significant feeding difficulties; disturbances of oral pharyngeal reflexes due to prolonged intubation may account for this. Other complicating nutritional factors may include aspiration during swallowing, gastroesophageal reflux, rumination, or necrotizing enterocolitis. Recurrent aspiration can complicate BPD, causing failure to recover. In infants with these problems, there may be a dramatic improvement after recognition and appropriate medical or surgical therapy. Some infants require nasogastric feedings or gastrostomy tubes (see Chapter 5).

Poor growth is common in these infants. They often require 30–50 percent more calories than infants without BPD to achieve normal growth rates. Their metabolic rates are somewhat increased, but the breathing work of the ventilatory muscles alone does not account for this.[33,34] Also, treatment with

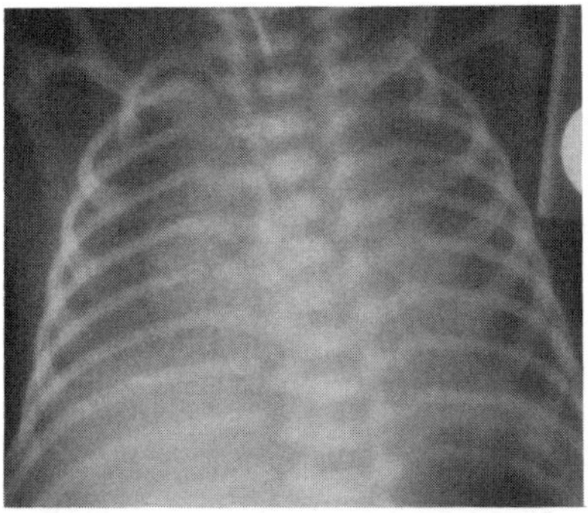

**FIGURE 2 ■ Radiograph of a 1,000 gm, 29 week infant on the first day of life.** It shows generalized reticular granular density throughout both lungs characteristic of respiratory distress syndrome.

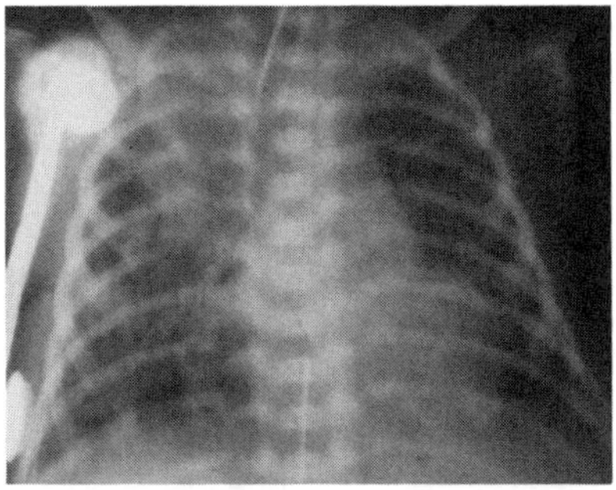

**FIGURE 3 ■ Same infant on the ninth day of life.** There is widespread patchy and streaky densities throughout the lungs. Also noted is increased lung density due to a combination of underaeration and edema.

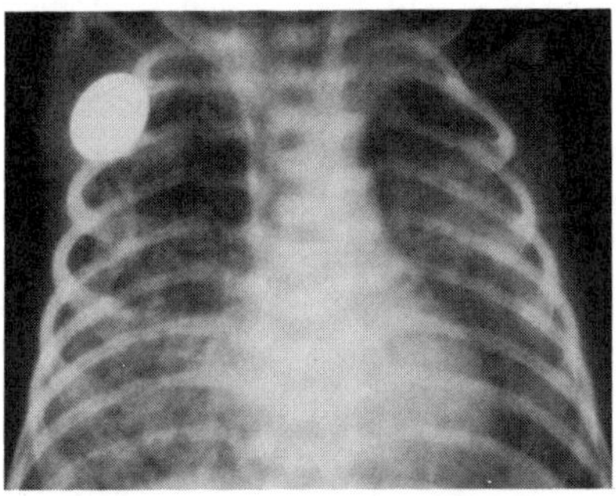

**FIGURE 4 ■ By the 20th day of life,** this infant has radiographic findings consistent with persistent moderate to severe bronchopulmonary dysplasia, including evidence of fibrosis and cystic changes.

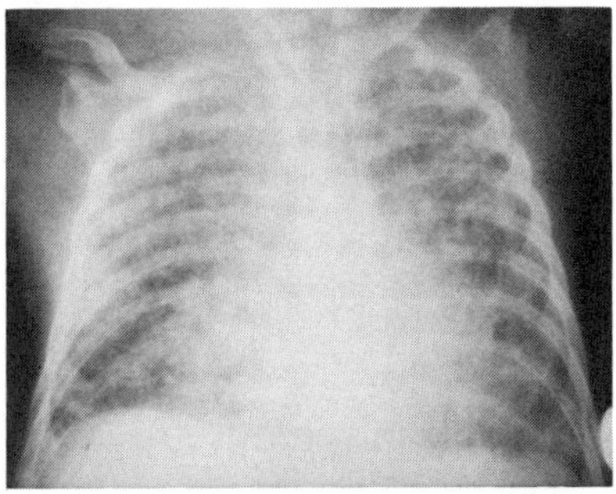

**FIGURE 5 ■ On the 75th day of life,** this infant has severe BPD with increased density of lungs and focal areas of pseudocystic changes in the right and left midlung fields. This infant had very severe BPD necessitating a tracheostomy at six months for mechanical ventilation lasting over a year.

diuretics or bronchodilators, which decrease the work of breathing substantially, does not decrease the metabolic rate in these infants.[35] The energy required by chronic inflammation and the pulmonary repair processes may better account for these increased metabolic demands.

Tracheal stenosis is a severe complication of chronic intubation in these infants. They may have areas of subglottic scarring due to tracheal trauma, pressure necrosis, and tracheitis.[36,37] A tracheostomy can greatly facilitate care, allow greater mobility, and increase comfort in infants who are chronically ventilator dependent. However, tracheostomy in a young infant also carries a substantial long-term morbidity and mortality.

Cor pulmonale is a common but usually preventable complication of BPD. Chronic or intermittent hypoxemia may lead to right and left ventricular hypertrophy.[38,39] Adequate oxygenation may be difficult to achieve because these infants can be quite labile. Also, the pain associated with arterial sampling can affect oxygenation. Transcutaneous oxygen levels, useful in acute respiratory management of premature infants, do not accurately measure arterial oxygen levels in infants with BPD who are 8 to 12 weeks old, probably due to increasing thickness of the epidermal layer.[40] Maintaining an infant's oxygen saturation *consistently* greater than or equal to 92 percent prevents the development of cor pulmonale. If cor pulmonale with heart failure does develop (usually as a result of an acute viral respiratory infection), the infant will often require mechanical ventilation and chronic therapy for many months.

Another complication of BPD is osteopenia.[41] Because calcium deposition normally occurs during the last two months of gestation and calcium supplementation is difficult in these infants, osteopenia or rickets may result. Vitamin D deficiency and use of potent diuretics can also predispose the infant to these changes. Chest radiograms may show a decreased degree of bone density. In severe cases, multiple rib and long bone fractures may develop. (These complications are further elaborated in Chapter 3.)

## Therapy

Judicious use of oxygen, mechanical ventilation, and fluid and nutritional therapy are cornerstones in the treatment of infants with BPD. Drug therapy remains controversial. Because infants with bronchopulmonary dysplasia have interstitial pulmonary edema, treatment with diuretics has been used for many years. Initially, diuretics were used empirically; their use has recently been substantiated by objective studies. Using an infant body plethysmograph to measure pulmonary function, researchers demonstrated that intravenous furosemide results in a prompt, dramatic decrease in airway resistance, which returns to baseline after 4–6 hours. Dynamic compliance shows a similar improvement. Lung volume, however, does not change.[42] Therapy with oral furosemide has been disappointing because its absorption in neonates is irregular.[43] Oral therapy with chorothiazide (Diuril), however, does result in improved airway resistance and dynamic compliance similar to that of intravenous furosemide.[44]

The use of bronchodilators was controversial before appropriate techniques were developed to objectively measure pulmonary function in infants. Because normal infants have little peribronchial smooth muscle, many pediatricians were reluctant to use bronchodilators. However, a remarkable hypertrophy of peribronchial smooth muscle has been found on autopsy of infants with terminal BPD, even at a young age. Investigators have demonstrated that the use of aerosolized isoproterenol promptly improves airway resistance.[45] When suitable techniques were developed for studying pulmonary function in infants on ventilators, researchers were able to demonstrate the development of responsiveness to bronchodilators by three weeks of age in premature infants with respiratory failure.[29,30] One hypothesis is that the development of peribronchial smooth muscle hypertrophy is a nonspecific response to lung injury.

The use of methylxanthines is more controversial. Until the development of adequate microtechniques to measure the pharmacokinetics of methylxanthines, they were considered unsafe in infants. The clearance of methylxanthines is slow in young infants. Also, individual infants react very differently to medication, and the metabolism may change dramatically as the liver matures.

An appropriate starting dosage for theophylline in infants less than one year of age can be calculated using the following formula:

*8 + age in months = daily dosage in mg per kg*[46]

Blood levels should then be checked and the dosage adjusted accordingly. Because the half-life of theophylline may be 24 hours or longer in young premature infants, dosing intervals may be extended.

It has been demonstrated that theophylline improves airway resistance, dynamic compliance, and flow at functional residual capacity.[47] In addition to the improvement of respiratory mechanics, methylxanthines also improve central ventilatory drive and may improve ventilatory muscle contractility.[48,49]

Weaning infants with BPD from ventilatory support is often difficult. Generally, infants with chronic respiratory failure cannot be weaned from the ventilator until they are provided with adequate calories for positive nitrogen balance.[50] In my experience, weaning can be safely accomplished even when infants cannot maintain a normal carbon dioxide level, as long as they have a compensatory metabolic alkalosis so that their pH remains normal. This minimizes the degree of airway trauma from the ventilator and may allow for further lung recovery at a faster rate.

A few infants are particularly difficult to wean from the ventilator. They often are able to make gradual progress interrupted by dramatic setbacks requiring increased ventilator rate, pressure, and $FiO_2$. In some of these infants, episodes of deterioration are due to ventilatory muscle fatigue. These infants may be successfully weaned by conditioning their ventilatory muscles by using short periods of ventilation with low rates, then longer periods of rest with increased rates utilizing the ventilator to do the work of breathing. Using this conditioning technique, some infants can gradually take over the work of breathing and be successfully weaned. This method has been effective in infants who have been ventilator dependent for more than a year and may have merit in younger infants in whom conventional weaning techniques have been unsuccessful.

## Family Care

The families of all infants with BPD undergo severe emotional trauma. The experience of dealing with a pregnancy complicated by premature delivery followed by the distress engendered by having an extremely sick infant hospitalized for prolonged periods of time, often with alternating slow improvement and sudden severe setbacks, is traumatic to the most emotionally robust families. The mandates of critical care with invasive treatment and monitoring obstruct effective parent-infant bonding. Parents and family members feel unwelcome and in the way in busy, noisy, crowded intensive care units with their frequent loud alarms, strict handwashing and gown-wearing regimens, and stressed staff who use unfamiliar technical jargon. Because of the regionalization of neonatal intensive care, many parents are forced to travel long distances to visit their infants. The financial burdens to families of infants with severe BPD, whose medical bills often exceed a hundred thousand dollars, add to their other stresses.

Infants with BPD are often born to women who lack the social support of an extended family and who have not had prenatal care. Thus, mothers who have had very little contact with the medical care system find themselves with an infant with extremely complex and critical medical needs. Infants with BPD are frequently ready for discharge before their families are ready to handle their care. More and earlier attention to the support of families of infants with this disease is essential.

## Discharge and Home Care

Discharge of infants with BPD from the hospital is becoming a more important issue as cost constraints increase. Often these infants are clinically unstable, with dramatic changes in their respiratory status, which then affect other systems. Their oxygen requirements and need for medications and frequent monitoring may change dramatically. Infants with severe BPD may need management in the hospital for long periods of time even when they do not require intubation. However, many infants may be discharged home if they have capable caretakers and adequate home equipment and if appropriate nursing relief for families can be provided. If this is done judiciously, prolonged hospitalization can be reduced. However, the costs of home nursing are also great, and home nursing can be difficult to withdraw from families who come to depend on it (see Chapter 9).

After these infants are discharged from the hospital, they often improve dramatically. As the infant becomes more stable, the fluctuations in respiratory status decrease. Weight gain is frequently achieved more easily. (Failure to gain weight at 15–30 gm per day at home is a poor prognostic sign and warrants more aggressive therapy with increased calories and a close look at $FiO_2$ levels.) The infant may devote more energy to social and developmental skills. Because the infant is usually exposed to fewer caretakers in the home environment, upper respiratory infections become less frequent.

Despite these improvements, the rate of rehospitalization of these infants is substantial. Infants with BPD display a high incidence of unexpected death. Some of them are classified as having sudden infant death syndrome, although the pathophysiologic mechanisms might be different from those in the majority of SIDS victims who were previously healthy. The use of home apnea and bradycardia monitors in infants with BPD is still controversial.

Viral upper-respiratory infections with respiratory syncytial virus, adenovirus, influenza, parainfluenza, and others are major risks for infants with BPD. Not infrequently, chronically hospitalized infants will be subjected to recurrent infections with respiratory syncytial virus, which is passed from infant to infant by fomites and staff. These infants frequently develop severe respiratory manifestations with wheezing, tachypnea, and hypoxia and require prolonged periods of mechanical ventilation. Chronic use of diuretics may decrease the risk of rehospitalization, but this has not yet been demonstrated by controlled clinical trials.

Systolic hypertension is a common complication in infants with BPD.[51] It may result from pharmacologic therapy or may be idiopathic. Therapy with antihypertensive medications may be required.

Generally, infants with BPD gradually improve during the first two years of life, probably due to the effects of rapid alveolar growth and gradual repair of damaged airways. Many of these infants have a good long-term prognosis. However, they continue to have reversible airway obstruction episodes of wheezing during upper respiratory infections or following vigorous exercise. Their pulmonary function remains abnormal, with follow-up studies indicating gas trapping and decreased small airway function. A study of the exercise performance of school-age children who had required mechanical ventilation

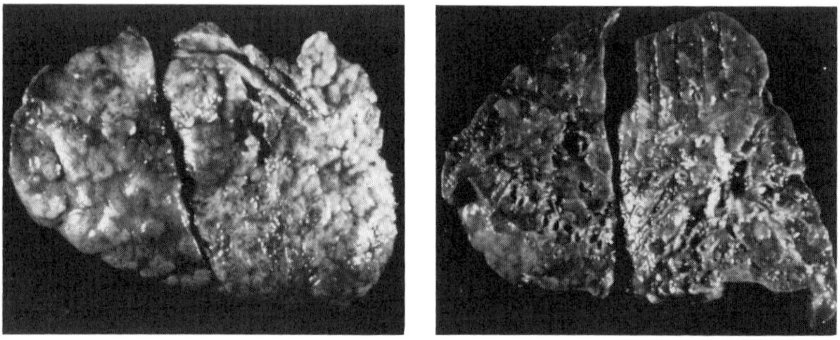

**FIGURES 6 & 7 ■ Whole lung and cut surface showing bronchopulmonary dysplasia stage IV** with alternating zones of hyperinflation and altelectasis.

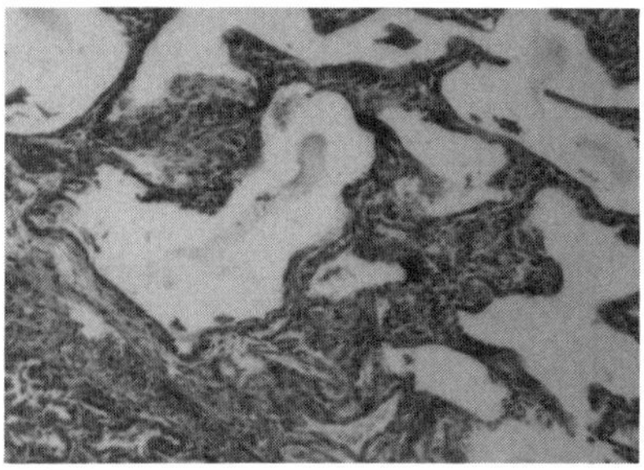

**FIGURE 8 ■ Photomicrograph showing** (a) area of hyperinflation, and (b) cystic remodeling of alveoli adjacent to area of hyperinflation.

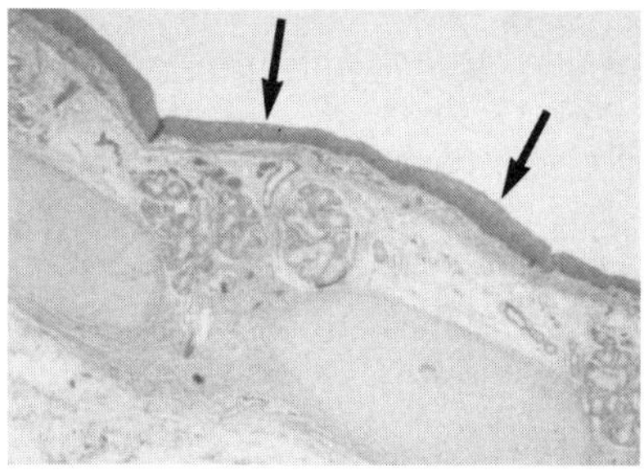

**FIGURE 9 ■ Longitudinal section of trachea in an infant with BPD.** Arrows indicate squamous metaplasia.

Courtesy of Roger Williams, MD, Chief of Pathology, Children's Hospital, Oakland, California.

as neonates showed that 3 of 20 subjects experienced inappropriate carbon dioxide retention during vigorous exercise.[52] A study of nine children aged 7 to 9 who had BPD in infancy demonstrated that their spirometry, lung volumes, and bronchio-reactivity tests remained abnormal.

For some infants, however, BPD progresses to terminal respiratory failure at some time during the first year of life. It is difficult to identify this group of infants during the first few weeks of hospitalization, but in retrospect their early courses are marked by very severe acute lung disease, and later complicated by infections and unstable clinical parameters. Figures 6 through 9 illustrate several aspects of pulmonary pathology seen on autopsy of infants who have died from respiratory failure secondary to BPD.

## Summary

Bronchopulmonary dysplasia is a common sequel of respiratory disease in the neonatal period. Pulmonary damage caused by oxygen toxicity, barotrauma, and inflammatory insults to the lungs are the major etiologic factors. Therapy requires meticulous respiratory, nutritional, and social intervention. Infants with BPD continue to require frequent medical care for the first 2–3 years of life and have demonstrable respiratory function abnormalities in middle childhood.

## References

1. Northway WH, Rosan RC, and Porter DY: Pulmonary disease following respiratory therapy for hyaline membrane disease; bronchopulmonary dysplasia, New England Journal of Medicine 276, 1967, pp. 357–368.
2. Northway WH: Observations on bronchopulmonary dysplasia, Journal of Pediatrics 95, 1979, pp. 815–818.
3. Saugstad OD: Oxygen radicals and pulmonary damage, Pediatric Pulmonology 1, 1985, pp. 167–175.
4. Smith TC, Gross JB, and Wollman H: The therapeutic gases oxygen, carbon dioxide, helium, and water vapor, *in* Gilman AG, et al., eds., Goodman and Gilman's Pharmacological Basis of Therapeutics, 7th ed., New York, 1985, Macmillan.
5. Miller JW, and Winter PM: Clinical manifestations of pulmonary oxygen toxicity, International Anesthesiology Clinics 19, 1981, pp. 179–199.
6. Deneke SM, and Fanburg BL: Normobaric oxygen toxicity to the lung, New England Journal of Medicine 303, 1980, pp. 76–86.
7. Reynolds EOR, and Taghizadeh A: Improved prognosis of infants mechanically ventilated for hyaline membrane disease, Archives of Disease in Childhood 49, 1974, pp. 505–515.
8. Taghizadeh A, and Reynolds EOR: Pathogenesis of bronchopulmonary dysplasia following hyaline membrane disease, American Journal of Pathology 82, 1976, p. 241.
9. Moylan FMB, et al.: Alveolar rupture as an independent predictor of bronchopulmonary dysplasia, Critical Care Medicine 6, 1978, pp. 10–13.
10. Moyland FMB, et al.: The relationship of bronchopulmonary dysplasia to the occurrence of alveolar rupture during positive pressure ventilation, Critical Care Medicine 6, 1978, pp. 140–142.
11. Rhodes PG, et al.: Minimizing pneumothorax and bronchopulmonary dysplasia in ventilated infants with hyaline membrane disease, Journal of Pediatrics 103, 1983, pp. 634–637.
12. Berg TJ, et al.: Bronchopulmonary dysplasia and lung rupture in hyaline membrane disease: Influence of continuous distending pressure, Pediatrics 55, 1975, pp. 51–54
13. Froese AB, and Bryan AC: High frequency ventilation state of the art, American Review of Respiratory Disease 135, 1987, pp. 1363–1374.
14. Marchak BE, et al.: Treatment of RDS by high-frequency oscillatory ventilation: A preliminary report, Journal of Pediatrics 99, 1981, p. 292.

15. Boros SJ, et al.: Neonatal high-frequency jet ventilation: Four years experience, Pediatrics 75, 1985, pp. 657–663.
16. Gay JH, Daily WJR, and Meyer BHP: Ligation of the patent ductus arteriosus in premature infants: Report of 45 cases, Journal of Pediatric Surgery 8, 1973, pp. 677–683.
17. Brown ER, et al.: Bronchopulmonary dysplasia: Possible relationship to pulmonary edema, Journal of Pediatrics 92, 1978, pp. 982–984.
18. Coates AL, et al.: Long-term pulmonary sequelae of premature birth with and without idiopathic respiratory distress syndrome, Journal of Pediatrics 90, 1977, pp. 611–616.
19. Taussig LM: Clinical and physiologic evidence for the persistence of pulmonary abnormalities after respiratory illnesses in infancy and childhood, Pediatric Research 11, 1977, pp. 216-218.
20. Burrows B, Knudson RJ, and Lebowitz MD: The relationship of childhood respiratory illness to adult obstructive airway disease, American Review of Respiratory Disease 115, 1977, pp. 751–760.
21. Kattan M, et al.: Pulmonary function abnormalities in symptom-free children after bronchiolitis, Pediatrics 59, 1977, pp. 683–688.
22. Sims DG, et al.: Study of 8-year-old children with a history of respiratory syncytial virus bronchiolitis in infancy, British Medical Journal I, 1978, pp. 11–14.
23. Loughlin GM, and Taussig LM: Pulmonary function in children with a history of laryngotracheobronchitis, Journal of Pediatrics 94, 1979, pp. 365–369.
24. Yahav J, Lieberman P, and Molho M: Pulmonary function following the adult respiratory distress syndrome, Chest 74, 1978, pp. 247–250.
25. Elliott CG, Morris AH, and Cengiz M: Pulmonary function and exercise gas exchange in survivors of adult respiratory distress syndrome, American Review of Respiratory Disease 123, 1981, pp. 492–495.
26. Churg A, et al.: Bronchopulmonary dysplasia in the adult, American Review of Respiratory Diseases 127, 1983, pp. 117–120.
27. Nickerson BF, and Taussig LM: Family history of asthma in infants with bronchopulmonary dysplasia, Pediatrics 65, 1980, pp. 1140–1144.
28. Belik J, et al.: Effect of early furosemide administration in neonates with respiratory distress syndrome, Pediatric Pulmonology 3, 1987, pp. 219–225.
29. Motayama EK, et al.: Early onset of airway reactivity in premature infants with bronchopulmonary dysplasia, American Review of Respiratory Diseases 136, 1987, pp. 50–57.
30. Sosulski R, et al.: Physiological effects of terbutaline on pulmonology function of infants with bronchopulmonary dysplasia, Pediatric Pulmonology 2, 1986, pp. 269–273.
31. Merritt TA, et al.: Newborn tracheal aspirate cytology: Classification during respiratory distress syndrome and bronchopulmonary dysplasia, Journal of Pediatrics 98, 1981, pp. 949–956.
32. Ogden BE, et al.: Lung lavage of newborns with respiratory distress syndrome, Chest 83, 1983, pp. 331S–333S.
33. Weinstein MR, and Oh W: Oxygen consumption in infants with bronchopulmonary dysplasia, Journal of Pediatrics 99, 1981, pp. 958–960.

34. Wolfson MR, et al.: Mechanics and energetics of breathing helium in infants with bronchopulmonary dysplasia, Journal of Pediatrics 104, 1984, pp. 752–757.
35. Kao LC, Durand DJ, and Nickerson BG: Improving pulmonary function does not decrease oxygen consumption in infants with bronchopulmonary dysplasia, Journal of Pediatrics 111, 1987, pp. 439–444.
36. Rasche RFH, and Kuhns LR: Histopathologic changes in airway mucosa of infants after endotracheal intubation, Pediatrics 50, 1972, pp. 632–637.
37. Mann DG, and Kirchner JA: Bronchopulmonary dysplasia (or subglottic stenosis?), Laryngoscope 92, 1982, pp. 976–979.
38. Melnick G, et al.: Normal pulmonary vascular resistance and left ventricular hypertrophy in young infants with bronchopulmonary dysplasia: An echocardiographic and pathologic study, Pediatrics 66, 1980, pp. 589–596.
39. Berman W, et al.: Evaluation of infants with bronchopulmonary dysplasia using cardiac catheterization, Pediatrics 70, 1982, pp. 708–712.
40. Rome ES, et al.: Limitations of transcutaneous $PO_2$ and $PCO_2$ monitoring in infants with bronchopulmonary dysplasia, Pediatrics 74, 1984, pp. 217–220.
41. Venkataraman PS, et al.: Secondary hyperparathyroidism and bone disease in infants receiving long-term furosemide therapy, American Journal of Diseases of Children 137, 1983, pp. 1158–1181.
42. Kao LC, et al.: Furosemide acutely decreases airways resistance in chronic bronchopulmonary dysplasia, Journal of Pediatrics 103, 1983, pp. 624–629.
43. Peterson RG, et al.: Pharmacology of furosemide in the premature newborn infant, Journal of Pediatrics 97, 1980, pp. 139–143.
44. Kao LC, et al.: Effect of oral diuretics on pulmonary mechanics in infants with chronic bronchopulmonary dysplasia: Results of a double-blind crossover sequential trial, Pediatrics 74, 1984, pp. 37–44.
45. Kao LC, et al.: Effect of isoproterenol inhalation on airway resistance in chronic bronchopulmonary dysplasia, Pediatrics 73, 1984, pp. 509–513.
46. Nassif EG, et al.: Theophylline disposition in infancy, Journal of Pediatrics 98, 1981, pp. 158–161.
47. Kao LC, et al.: Oral theophylline and diuretics improve pulmonary mechanics in infants with bronchopulmonary dysplasia, Journal of Pediatrics 111, 1987, pp. 439–444.
48. Harris MC, et al.: Successful extubation of infants with respiratory distress syndrome using aminophylline, Journal of Pediatrics 103, 1983, pp. 303–305.
49. Aubier M. et al.: Aminophylline improves diaphragmatic contractility, New England Journal of Medicine 305, 1982, pp. 240–246.
50. Morray JP, et al.: Clinical correlates of successful weaning from mechanical ventilation in severe bronchopulmonary dysplasia, Critical Care 9, 1981, pp. 815–818.
51. Heldt GP, et al.: Exercise performance of the survivors of hyaline membrane disease, Journal of Pediatrics 96, 1980, pp. 995–999.
52. Abaman SH, et al.: Systemic hypertension in infants with bronchopulmonary dysplasia, Journal of Pediatrics 104, 1984, pp. 928–931.

CHAPTER 2

# Respiratory Management of the Infant with BPD

*Rosalyn Feller Scherf, RNC*
*Northshore Medical Center Hospital*
*Miami, Florida*

The keys to respiratory management of infants with BPD are patience and consistency. Management of these infants can be frustrating and tedious. Frequently, progress is made, only to be followed by failure and regression. Prolonged hospitalization, pulmonary morbidity, and other serious complications mark the course of this disease, and pulmonary complications create obstacles such as prolonged oxygen and/or ventilatory dependency that are difficult to surmount.

These infants are in varying degrees of respiratory failure. Attempts to maintain adequate tissue oxygenation and alveolar ventilation are hindered by the presence of hypoxemia and hypercapnia (carbon dioxide retention).[1] These two conditions make respiratory management difficult and can impede efforts to wean these infants from their respiratory support.

Weaning babies from the ventilator and/or oxygen support should be attempted on a regular, consistent basis as long as the infant is not acutely ill (as with a respiratory infection).[2] The weaning process has to be done slowly, in small increments.[1–4] In many cases, the lungs will improve with time as a result of the normal growth and repair process.[5] These improvements occur over long periods of time—sometimes weeks to months. Pulmonary function tests on infants with appropriate weight gain show gradual increases in lung compliance, decreases in airway resistance and respiratory effort, and improvement in functional residual capacity (FRC).[3,6,7] It is therefore essential that nutritional needs are adequately met to enable these infants to grow.[3,6] (The role of nutrition is discussed in Chapter 5.)

It is extremely important that the medical, nursing, respiratory and developmental team are in agreement with the established plan of care developed for each infant. This will provide the consistency and continuity of care that is so vital.

Although respiratory management has to be tailored individually, there are some generalized principles and guidelines of care. This chapter reviews these principles and guidelines as they apply to the hospitalized, ventilator-dependent infant with BPD as well as the extubated infant who is still oxygen dependent.

## Oxygenation

Because of changes in lung tissue, infants with BPD are oxygen dependent.[1,6,8] Inflammation and destruction of the alveolar wall or of its capillary bed cause a destructive form of emphysema. A diffusion barrier is created with collapse of some alveoli and overdistension of others. Pulmonary function tests show a decrease in dynamic lung compliance, an increase in airway resistance, and an increase in the work (or effort) of breathing. FRC may be decreased, increased, or, in some cases, even normal.[1,3,6]

Infants with BPD are already utilizing their maximum capacity to maintain respiratory function. It takes very little stress to cause them to decompensate and become hypoxic and/or more hypercapnic. All these existing conditions make it difficult or impossible to decrease their fraction of inspired oxygen ($FiO_2$) or wean them from their ventilatory support.

It is important to prevent hypoxemia and hypercapnia even when minimal ventilatory support that avoids further destruction of lung tissue is the goal. Echocardiographic studies have shown that as long as arterial oxygen tension ($PaO_2$) is maintained above 55 mmHg, pulmonary artery pressures are normal.[1,9-11] Maintaining this $PaO_2$ may prevent pulmonary hypertension and its additional complications such as right ventricular failure and, eventually, cor pulmonale. This is particularly important for an infant who is showing clinical signs of a patent ductus arteriosus (PDA) and/or pulmonary hypertension. Maintaining $PaO_2$ at 55 mmHg or above may prevent further respiratory decompensation and lessen the degree of pulmonary hypertension, resulting in improved oxygenation and ventilation.[1,8-11]

**Interventions for Assessing and Improving Oxygenation**

1. Maintain required $FiO_2$ at all times, especially during periods of stress, as when suctioning or starting an IV. Even routine daily care like weighing, bathing, and feeding can be very stressful.[1,12–15] Oxygen consumption increases during feedings and in the presence of hypothermia. This may cause the $PaO_2$ to decrease. Therefore, it may be necessary to increase $FiO_2$ during feedings or during procedures that might cause hypothermia, such as bathing.
2. Monitor the infant's oxygenation by using transcutaneous oxygen tension ($TcPO_2$) or pulse oximetry ($SaO_2$) to determine each infant's pattern (or degree of stress) during some procedures.[7,13,16] Ventilator and oxygen changes can be made if necessary. If a pattern of hypoxia is detected and an increase in settings is ordered during procedures such as suctioning, the infant should be periodically re-evaluated to see if this increase is still necessary. As the infant's lungs improve, both the episodes of hypoxia and the need for increased support during procedures should lessen.

   Transcutaneous monitors and pulse oximeters are the methods to monitor a patient's response to different levels of activities and to various procedures. Several studies have found limitations, however, in using transcutaneous monitoring on older infants, including underestimation of arterial $PO_2$.[17,18] This is because of the changes in skin thickness in the older infants with BPD. A differing result was reported by Satish and Douglas, who found that transcutaneous monitoring can be a valuable tool in managing BPD infants,[19] if oxygenation trends are utilized and not exact figures.

   Pulse oximetry has recently been examined as an alternative method of monitoring oxygen status in infants with both acute and chronic respiratory disease. In two recent studies, improved assessment of oxygenation was obtained with pulse oximetry monitoring than with transcutaneous monitoring, as long as saturation levels were greater than 78 percent.[20,21] The primary limitation encountered with pulse oximetry was sensitivity to motion artifact. This may be reduced by setting the sensitivity on the pulse oximeter at a slightly lower level.[20]
3. If an infant tends to readily become cyanotic and hypoxic during periods of stress, increasing the current $FiO_2$ by 5–10 percent immediately before doing a procedure such as suctioning might alleviate the severity of hypoxia or help maintain adequate oxygenation, and thus completely prevent hypoxic episodes.[12,15,22] Five to ten minutes after the procedure, decrease the $FiO_2$ to the previous concentration in one or two steps to prevent hyperoxia.

**TABLE 1 ■ Acidosis and its Effect on Various Body Systems**

***Respiratory system***

- Shifts oxygen-hemoglobin dissociation curve to the right, resulting in a higher $PaO_2$ being necessary to produce a given oxygen saturation
- Increases pulmonary artery pressure, causes pulmonary arterial vasoconstriction:
  - Has a synergistic effect with hypoxia if the pH is above 7.1
  - Has an independent effect if the pH is 7.1 or lower
- May result in ventilation-perfusion abnormalities
- Interferes with surfactant production

***Cardiovascular system***

- If severe, dramatically depresses cardiac function:
  - Decreases myocardial contractility
  - Decreases coronary blood flow
  - Interferes with myocardial uptake of glucose
  - Affects cell membrane potential
  - Lowers threshold for ventricular fibrillation
- Circulation is refractory to sympathomimetic amines

***Central nervous system***

- Depresses CNS causing:
  - Headache
  - Lethargy
  - Confusion
  - Coma

***Blood chemistry***

- Hyperkalemia. Potassium tends to leave intracellular compartment, which raises myocardial cell membrane potentials, slowing the heart rate and leading to asystole
- Hyperbilirubinemia-kernicterus. May diminish the binding of bilirubin by albumin, thereby enhancing the development of kernicterus
- Hypocalcemia. May decrease the force of myocardial contraction

***Miscellaneous***

- With late metabolic acidosis, infants do not gain weight as rapidly (it is questionable if this effect is primary or secondary)

4. Measurements of arterial and/or capillary blood gases are done according to each unit's established guidelines or protocols. For example, in some units blood gases are obtained every three days and also usually 20 minutes after a permanent change in $FiO_2$ or ventilator settings. If the infant shows signs of distress, such as increased respiratory rate, increased heart rate, cyanosis, increased retractions, rales, lethargy, or increased oxygen or ventilatory requirements, blood gases should be obtained more frequently.

Maintain $PaO_2$ and arterial carbon dioxide tension ($PaCO_2$) within normal acceptable limits: arterial $PaO_2$ 50–70 mmHg (or in some cases, 80 mmHg) and capillary $PaO_2$, 40–60 mmHg.[4,19] These ranges give flexibility to treat each individual infant. For example, an infant with multiple problems (failure to gain weight, anemia, or cor pulmonale) might require a $PaO_2$ of 60–70 or even 80 mmHg.

Acceptable limits for arterial $PaCO_2$ are 45–60 mmHg (normal $PaCO_2$ is 35–45 mmHg).[1,4,23] In some cases, higher $PaCO_2$ levels may be acceptable—this is individualized and depends on each infant's degree of illness. Some infants can have a $PaCO_2$ reading in the high 60s or low 70s and continue to be weaned from the ventilator—or even remain extubated. Their pH, base excess, and sodium bicarbonate levels must also be taken into consideration.

Some of these infants compensate fairly well and tolerate their elevated $PaCO_2$ levels. Nevertheless, their range of tolerance is minimal. Stressful episodes that are not readily corrected could cause them to decompensate rapidly. Acidosis can have serious effects on many body systems (Table 1). It should be readily treated (usually by increasing ventilator settings) when detected.

5. Decrease $FiO_2$, intermittent mandatory ventilation (IMV) rate, and peak inspiratory pressure (PIP) very slowly. These infants generally do not tolerate large decreases in their ventilatory settings. Reduction of $FiO_2$ by as little as 2 percent may result in hypoxia.[1,3,24] The same is true of reductions in the IMV rate and PIP. However, it is still important to wean on a regular schedule.[2]
6. Attempt to reduce episodes of agitation and crying. If the ventilated infant "fights" the ventilation provided, a pneumothorax is a potential complication. For the extubated infant, crying may help re-expand some atelectatic areas, but prolonged crying can result in cyanosis, hypoxia, and a decrease in ventilation. Hypoxia may become so severe that the infant decompensates to the point of requiring reintubation to restabilize his respiratory function. (To decompensate in this context means to become agitated, hypoxic, cyanotic, acidotic, lethargic, or hypercapnic and to develop air hunger.) It has frequently been observed in the clinical situation that a chronic lung patient who is reintubated for respiratory failure and placed back on mechanical ventilation can be very difficult to wean again from ventilatory support.
   a. Communicate clearly to other caregivers (in a care plan) whatever you've discovered calms the infant—rubbing his head, putting him on his abdomen or back, swaddling him, playing a tape recorder.

b. Consider temporarily increasing $FiO_2$ or ventilator settings during episodes of agitation. Some agitation can be the direct result of hypoxia and underventilation (i.e. "air hunger").
c. Sedation with medications such as chloral hydrate or phenobarbital may need to be given on a routine basis if the infant is very agitated.[4,23] Reevaluate the infant every four to seven days so these drugs can be discontinued as soon as possible. (See Chapter 4.)

7. Maintain an adequate hematocrit (30–40 percent) to provide the infant with optimum oxygen carrying capacity.[23] Administer blood transfusions over three to four hours to prevent fluid overload and resulting pulmonary edema.
8. For the older, extubated, but still oxygen-dependent infant, an oxygen source other than a plexiglass hood should be available. A nasal cannula is usually used in infants receiving 40 percent or less oxygen.
   a. During certain procedures such as bathing, feedings, and play periods, a nasal cannula enables the infant to have more normal contact with the environment and caretakers. The nasal cannula can give the older infant the freedom required to develop his gross motor and social skills.[13] Because exact concentrations of oxygen cannot be measured with the nasal cannula, the flow rate must be utilized instead.
   b. Some units deliver oxygen concentrations via cannula by hooking it onto a blender. Others run a 100 percent oxygen source only. Both methods require a flow meter and the use of $SaO_2$ or $TcPO_2$ monitoring, which determine the optimal flow rate for each infant. This flow rate can then be used as a baseline when employing the nasal cannula. If the infant becomes cyanotic, tachypneic, or has an increase in retractions, the flow can be increased.
   c. Oxygen tubing should be sufficiently long to allow the infant to move around. The cannulas generally have six feet of tubing; more can be added for older infants who are beginning to crawl, walk, or use a walker. The flow at the end of extended tubing should be adequate; the best way to be sure is to monitor the infant's oxygenation while using longer tubing.
   d. During nap periods and at night, a larger oxygen hood or tent may be fitted around the infant's chest, with his arms inside to allow him hand-to-mouth and hand-to-hand contact and to permit him to turn and move about more freely. Some units routinely switch from cannula to hood; others find the nasal cannula adequate at all times.
   e. Some infants weaned to room air might still require oxygen therapy at

night. Studies have shown that sleep is associated with alterations in lung mechanics, irregularity of breathing, and a fall in $PaO_2$.[25] To make sure he is not having hypoxic episodes, monitor $TcPO_2$ or $SaO_2$ while the infant is sleeping for several nights after he is weaned to room air.

## Ventilation

In the presence of chronic obstructive pulmonary disease, air enters the alveoli but cannot get out. Some alveoli become overdistended, other alveoli become airless and collapse, and pulmonary interstitial emphysema can develop.

The occurrence of atelectasis, plugging of the airways, and air trapping can lead to insufficient alveolar ventilation with consequent carbon dioxide retention. This is probably because of increased dead space ventilation resulting from a small tidal volume, which results from increasingly stiff and overdistended lungs.[26] The infant becomes tachypneic to compensate for the decrease in tidal volume. Increased airway resistance increases the work of breathing as the infant tries to overcome the resistance and stiffness of his poorly compliant lungs. Rales, intercostal and subcostal retractions, and nasal flaring can be present. Efforts must be made to decrease the infant's work of breathing and maintain adequate ventilation.

Various types of ventilators are available for treating respiratory failure in neonates. A time-cycled, pressure-limited ventilator delivers a set PIP, regardless of the lung compliance. This can be advantageous when an infant has a decrease in compliance and very stiff lungs, because the amount of pressure delivered to the lungs will be limited. These ventilators are used extensively in neonatal units. A disadvantage is that the preset PIP may be too high when the compliance of the infant is improving. The machine cannot detect a change in compliance and will not, therefore, automatically decrease the pressure delivered to the lungs. This can result in barotrauma and possible worsening of lung tissue damage.

A volume-cycled ventilator delivers a preset volume of gas instead of a preset PIP. Because pressures vary with changes in compliance, it is generally possible to achieve better oxygenation and ventilation. (Lung compliance determines how much pressure is needed to deliver a set volume.) The PIP adjusts to the patient's needs even as they change.

There are some disadvantages to using a volume ventilator. When compliance decreases, high pressures may be necessary to deliver the set volume of gas, and this may result in air trapping, impeding of venous return, hyperventilation and a decreased respiratory drive, and barotrauma with possible wors-

**TABLE 2 ■ Advantages and Disadvantages of Long-Term Endotracheal Intubation and Tracheostomy**

| LONG-TERM ENDOTRACHEAL INTUBATION | |
|---|---|
| ***Advantages*** | ***Disadvantages*** |
| No surgical procedure | Laryngeal edema/damage |
| No anesthesia required | Can result in subglottic stenosis |
| When assisted ventilation no longer needed, infant can vocalize normally | Unable to vocalize while intubated |
| Easier, safer discharge without tracheostomy | Unable to nipple feed |
| No scar on neck | Tube can slip into bronchus |
| | Constant tape to face/difficult to secure |
| | Need skilled person to replace ET tube/ usually an emergency situation |
| **TRACHEOSTOMY** | |
| ***Advantages*** | ***Disadvantages*** |
| No damage to larynx | Post-op: difficult to deliver high PIP because of air leak |
| Cannot slip into bronchus | Long-term commitment to trach (usually), even after assisted ventilation no longer needed (12–24 months) |
| No tape to face | Delays speech acquisition/patient usually unable to vocalize |
| Able to oral feed | Skin problems and infection at stoma site |
| Easily replaced if plugged or dislodged | Home care complicated: may require home nursing services; risk of trach plugging, death |
| Infant more easily held without risk of tube dislodging: better for infant development and parent interaction | Scar when removed |

ening of BPD. Also, infants usually have to weigh 3 kg or more before they can be ventilated with a volume ventilator.

Regardless of which ventilator is chosen to treat a specific patient, it should adequately oxygenate and ventilate the infant.

## Interventions for Decreasing or Minimizing Hypercapnia

1. Maintain a secure and patent airway.
   a. Make sure the extubated infant is properly positioned to avoid occluding trachea and nares. For example, do not leave the head in a flexed

position that places pressure on the trachea nor in a severely hyperextended position.

When a nasogastric tube is left in place, it partially occludes one nare. Extubated infants are nose breathers, and blocking one nare creates a partial obstruction of the airway. In general, it is best to avoid leaving a nasogastric tube in place; however, if the infant becomes greatly stressed by repeated gavage tube insertions, the decision to leave an indwelling nasogastric tube may be made. It is best to use the smallest possible nasogastric tube and try to pass it orally, instead of nasally.

When indicated, do nasal and/or tracheal suction gently and quickly according to the unit's suction protocol.

b. In an intubated infant, the endotracheal tube (ET tube) should be securely stabilized. A very active or agitated infant needs to be swaddled and occasionally restrained to prevent him from pulling out the tube.

An appropriately sized ET tube should also be used. When a positive pressure of 30 cm $H_2O$ is applied to the airway, an appropriately sized tube will leak. If no leak is noticed, the ET tube may be replaced with a smaller tube.[24] However, an ET tube that is too small results in inefficient ventilation. The size of the tube should be reevaluated frequently as the infant grows.

c. If the infant is going to be intubated for a prolonged period (several months), a tracheostomy is usually considered.[24] There is no rule about when a tracheostomy should be performed. Some units will perform a tracheostomy if an infant is ventilated more than two months; others will wait four to six months; still others will never perform a tracheostomy for the purpose of chronic ventilation. Regardless of which policy is followed, periodic assessment via bronchoscopy for airway damage secondary to prolonged intubation should be performed.[27] (See Table 2 for the advantages and disadvantages of long-term endotracheal intubation and tracheostomy.)

d. Some units will also change from an oral to a nasal ET tube after six weeks of intubation if there is a need for chronic ventilation. A nasal ET tube allows the infant to suck on a pacifier, especially during feedings, and is generally more comfortable for the infant.

e. Provide adequate humidity through the ventilatory system to prevent damage to the respiratory tract mucosa. A decrease in either temperature or relative humidity of inspired gas can impair airway epithelial ciliary activity. ET tubes and tracheostomies must remain patent. Hypoxic episodes usually occur whenever an ET tube or tracheostomy tube has to be changed because of plugging.

f. Adequately suction ET tubes and tracheostomy tubes as needed, but try to prevent hypoxic episodes during suctioning. A PRN schedule would be more beneficial than having the infant on a rigid one or two hourly suctioning protocol.

For the extubated infant, occasional deep endotracheal suctioning may be required to remove mucus plugs and help re-expand collapsed lobes.[3] This may recruit collapsed alveoli, improve ventilation, and thereby decrease an elevated $PaCO_2$, allowing the infant to remain extubated.

2. Postural drainage with chest physiotherapy (CPT) and vibration followed by suctioning should be done as needed to prevent atelectasis and pooling of secretions.[1,15,28,29] The frequency depends on each individual infant's response as well as the severity of the disease, presence of atelectasis, and degree of carbon dioxide retention shown by blood gases or $TcCO_2$ monitoring. Increases in respiratory rate, rales, mucus, agitation, lethargy, and unresolved or increasing atelectasis observed on x-rays indicate a need for initiating or increasing the frequency of CPT. Although important, CPT must not be done so frequently as to exhaust the infant or cause so much agitation or sleep deprivation that hypoxia and hypercapnia result.[15] CPT done every one to two hours for six to eight hours at a time can be exhausting for the infant. Adequate rest periods should be provided. The effectiveness of the CPT must be weighed against the degree of hypoxia and respiratory distress that occurs from doing it.[12,15]

When atelectasis is present, the affected areas should be identified on the care plan so more effort is concentrated at those points. Handbagging the extubated infant after CPT for two to five minutes may also help to decrease an extremely elevated $PaCO_2$.[23]

3. For the intubated and ventilated infant on a time-cycled, pressure-limited ventilator, an IMV rate or PIP should be set to maintain the $PaCO_2$ in the high normal range (45–50 mmHg).[1,24] As mentioned previously, some units may accept a $PaCO_2$ in the 60–70 mmHg range if a normal pH is maintained. The lowest peak airway pressure and mean airway pressure (MAP) required to obtain adequate ventilation should be determined.[1] If the infant deteriorates, IMV, PIP, or both can be increased until the $PaCO_2$ has returned to *that infant's normal limits.* When increasing IMV, remember that the reduction of expiratory time below 0.5 seconds may produce air trapping. Venous return and cardiac output also may be affected.[30]

A positive end-expiratory pressure (PEEP) of 2–4 cm $H_2O$ can be used to stabilize lung volume by preventing the collapse of unstable alveoli. It can be adjusted so that the minimum oxygen concentration necessary is used to keep the $PaO_2$ at least 50–55 mmHg.

4. Medications such as bronchodilators, methylxanthines, diuretics, or steroids may be helpful in some infants.[7,31,32] Hypertrophy of peribronchiolar smooth muscle, an increase in airway resistance, and a decrease in compliance may warrant the use of a bronchodilator to lessen bronchospasm, decrease airway resistance, and improve lung mechanics.[7,15,31] Theophylline may be given to stimulate respiratory drive and aid in weaning from the ventilator.[1,4,7] Steroid therapy has been used successfully in some patients, but the risk of severe side effects, such as a decrease in resistance to infection, must be taken into consideration.[7]

   For infants with pulmonary edema or prominent rales, diuretics and/or fluid restriction have been used to decrease fluid retention and concurrently lower an elevated $PaCO_2$.[4,7,23,33] (Chapter 4 provides additional information on medications.)

5. For infants suffering from pulmonary edema or cor pulmonale, elevating the head of the bed may be helpful. Monitor fluids closely, and administer sedatives, digoxin, and diuretics as needed. Avoid stressing these infants: Allow them to rest as much as possible with minimal handling. Positioning the infant on his abdomen has been shown to improve oxygenation and ventilation.[34–37]

   For the intubated infant, in addition to the previously mentioned measures, increasing PEEP or continuous positive airway pressure settings might improve oxygenation and decrease the pulmonary edema by decreasing pulmonary blood flow. However, the increased PEEP might cause a rise in the $PaCO_2$. When normal alveoli become overdistended, their compliance decreases. This results in increased work of breathing, hypoventilation, and an increase in $PaCO_2$.

6. Remember basic principles such as stimulating the infant to cough and turning him frequently. These measures may help remove secretions, re-expand alveoli, and decrease $PaCO_2$.

7. In the presence of a lower respiratory tract infection, respiratory status decompensates even further. If this happens:
   a. Administer antibiotics as ordered by the physician.
   b. Increase CPT with suctioning if needed.
   c. Use extremely good handwashing techniques to prevent further cross-contamination.

**TABLE 3 ■ Examples of Weaning Schedules**

| | Monday | Tuesday | Wednesday | Thursday | Friday | Saturday | Sunday | Within 30 days it is possible to: |
|---|---|---|---|---|---|---|---|---|
| **Plan 1** | ↓$FiO_2$ by 1% | ↓$FiO_2$ by 1% & ↓PIP by 1 cm | ↓$FiO_2$ by 1% | ↓PIP by 1 cm | ↓$FiO_2$ by 1% | ↓IMV by 1 | ↓$FiO_2$ by 1% | ↓$FiO_2$ by 22%<br>↓IMV by 4 breaths<br>↓PIP by 9 cm |
| **Plan 2** | ↓$FiO_2$ by 1% | ↓$FiO_2$ by 1% & ↓IMV by 1 | ↓$FiO_2$ by 1% | ↓IMV by 1 & ↓PIP by 1 cm | No changes | ↓$FiO_2$ by 1% & ↓IMV by 1 | ↓$FiO_2$ by 1% & ↓PIP by 1 | ↓$FiO_2$ by 22%<br>↓IMV by 13 breaths<br>↓PIP by 8 cm |
| **Plan 3** | ↓$FiO_2$ by 1% | ↓IMV by 1 | ↓$FiO_2$ by 1% | No changes | ↓PIP by 1 cm | ↓$FiO_2$ by 1% | No changes | ↓$FiO_2$ by 13%<br>↓IMV by 5 breaths<br>↓PIP by 4 cm |
| **Plan 4** | ↓$FiO_2$ by 1% | ↓IMV by 1 | ↓$FiO_2$ by 1% | No changes | ↓$FiO_2$ by 1% | ↓$FiO_2$ by 1% | ↓IMV by 1 | ↓$FiO_2$ by 18%<br>↓IMV by 9 breaths<br>No change in PIP |

**WEANING PROCEDURE**

1. Wean as planned unless problems preventing or slowing weaning schedule arise.*
2. Allow at least 8 hours between changes on the same day.
3. When PIP setting is 18–22 cm, begin decreasing PEEP by 1 cm (every 1–2 days) until a PEEP of 2 cm is reached. (This is optional.)
4. Wean as tolerated by the infant but try to follow the plan.

* Examples of problems include: unexplained spontaneous bradycardia *(not* associated with suctioning), suspicion of respiratory infection, sepsis, NEC, severe carbon dioxide retention (the definition of severe is determined by each infant's individualized $PaCO_2$ pattern), signs of pulmonary edema, and continuous failure to have appropriate weight gain.

d. Avoid exposing the infant to caretakers and visitors with viral illnesses.

## Weaning

Clinical indications seen prior to successful weaning from mechanical ventilation have been identified and include a sustained decreasing trend in both $PaCO_2$ and respiratory rate, and improvement in weight gain pattern.[3] However, once these signs are present, it is important to proceed slowly and methodically as the infant gradually adjusts to the removal of mechanical ventilation. Weaning must be done *slowly* but *regularly*. These two points have purposely been mentioned several times. Their importance cannot be overemphasized.

It may seem ridiculous to wean these infants by only one percent $FiO_2$ or one increment of rate or PIP, but a significant amount of weaning can be accomplished in this way over a 30-day period. It is crucial that this be done on a regular schedule.[2,24] (Table 3) Depending on the infant's response, settings can be lowered every day or every second or third day—even on weekends and holidays.

A weaning schedule can be designed to accommodate each infant's specific problems. For example, if an infant has acceptable $PaCO_2$ levels but is on very high $FiO_2$ concentrations because of severe oxygen dependence, a plan to lower $FiO_2$ can be instituted. If the $FiO_2$ is low but ventilation (high $PaCO_2$) is a problem, then a plan to lower PIP and IMV can be instituted. If both oxygenation and ventilation are a problem, then a plan that *gradually* lowers $FiO_2$, IMV, and PIP can be developed.

In general, it is more advantageous to decrease settings slowly, by 1 percent a day to diminish the infant's response to decreased ventilatory support than to decrease them 5 percent in one day and then have the infant decompensate within 24–48 hours and require an increase in settings by 5–10 percent or more. When this pattern of "rapid" weaning has been observed in clinical practice, infants have regressed. (See Figure 1 for a comparison of a rapid weaning process and a slower method.)

The technique of plotting an infant's course was not developed as a method to institute "cookbook medicine." Its purpose is to serve as an example of a weaning care plan that can be individualized for every infant with BPD. It can be tailored to meet each infant's specific needs, whether it be oxygenation, ventilation, or both. In your unit, try making a graph similar to that shown in Figure 1 for any 30-day period of an infant with BPD. This may give you a picture of weaning trends in your unit.

For those babies who are difficult to wean from ventilation, Nickerson has described another method of weaning called sprinting.[38] This method is used in

**FIGURE 1 ■ Comparison Graph of Two Weaning Processes for a Ventilated Infant with BPD**

The black line graphs the actual amount of weaning done over a 30-day period by a typically stable infant with BPD. Very little was attempted or accomplished in regards to $FiO_2$. On day 7, IMV was increased for a few hours. On day 11, $FiO_2$ was decreased to 75 percent for a few hours, but the infant did not tolerate the 5 percent decrease and was placed back on 80 percent $FiO_2$. PIP was decreased for a few days. IMV eventually was decreased by four breaths, but PIP ultimately was increased to previous levels.

Superimposed (dotted line) is a graph of the progress made using the weaning process described in plan 3 of Table 3. A slower, methodical approach resulted in weaning the $FiO_2$ by 13 percent, the IMV rate by 5 breaths, and the PIP by 4 cm $H_2O$.

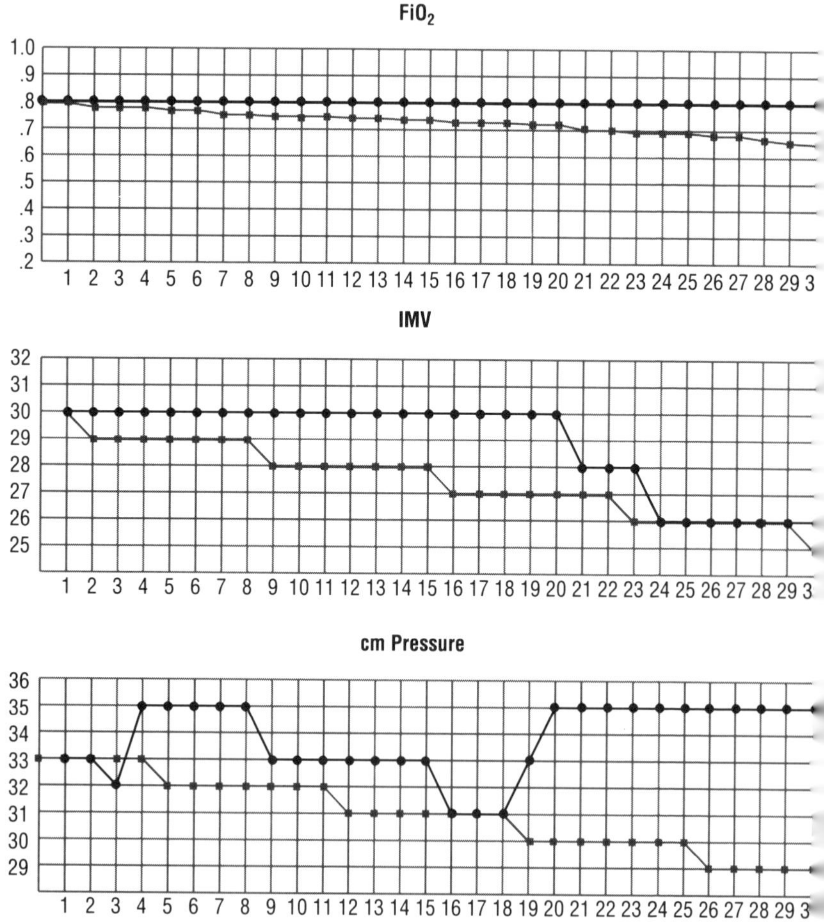

**TABLE 4 ■ Sprinting Method of Weaning**

SPRINT VENTILATOR SETTINGS (SAMPLE)

| *Usual Ventilator Settings* | *Sprinting Ventilator Settings* |
|---|---|
| $FiO_2$: 50% | $FiO_2$: 60% |
| PIP: 30/3 | PIP: 30/3 |
| Rate: 24 | Rate: 12 * |

*With ventilator rates less than 15, may consider sprinting to CPAP of 4–6 cm.

| *Schedule of Sprinting:* | *Record with each "Sprint":* |
|---|---|
| Day 1: Sprint 15 minutes each shift | a) $TcPO_2$ or $SaO_2$ trend |
| Day 3: Sprint 30 minutes each shift | b) Infant's respiratory effort |
| Day 7: Sprint 60 minutes each shift | c) Infant's behavioral state, any changes noted |
| Day 10: Sprint 1 1/4 hours each shift | d) Capillary blood gases obtained (if needed) at the end of the sprinting period |
| Day 15: Sprint 1 1/2 hours each shift | |
| Day 18: Sprint 1 3/4 hours each shift | |
| Day 21: Sprint 2 hours each shift | |
| Day 24: Sprint 2 1/2 hours each shift | |
| Day 27: Sprint 3 hours each shift | |
| Day 30: Sprint 4 hours each shift | |
| Day 35: Sprint 5 hours each shift | |
| Day 40: Sprint 6 hours each shift | |
| Day 45: Wean entirely to CPAP | |

infants whose inability to tolerate extubation may be due to fatigue of ventilatory muscles. Sprinting utilizes the principle that ventilatory muscular endurance must be increased in some infants before weaning can be successful. Periodic decreases in ventilatory support are followed by the infant's usual ventilatory support. (Table 4 shows an example of this approach.) This weaning method has proven successful in individual cases, but it should be further studied.

## Conclusion

Our main hope and encouragement in the care of neonates with respiratory diseases is to find precise ways to lessen the degree of BPD they may develop or to eliminate it entirely. All known factors that contribute to the development of BPD must be recognized quickly. Attempts can then be made to minimize these factors. The lowest mean airway pressures and oxygen concentration to provide adequate oxygenation and the lowest peak airway pressure required to obtain adequate ventilation should be used at all times, especially during the early stages of lung disease. In addition, as the mechanical characteristics of the lungs improve (such as an increase in compliance), both $FiO_2$ and pressure must be lowered rapidly to prevent damage to the lung.

As the course of BPD progresses, however, ventilatory management and respiratory care are somewhat different, as a slow, cautious weaning approach is adopted. The infant guides us through the process as we assess the markers of respiratory improvement: appropriate oxygenation and ventilation in all activities, as well as adequate somatic growth.

Thus, respiratory management of the infant with BPD remains a challenge that faces neonatal units. It is encouraging to know, however, that with appropriate weight gain, lung tissue does grow, and pulmonary function tests do improve.[3,6] In most cases, weaning from ventilatory support and oxygen is possible.

## Acknowledgement

The author gratefully acknowledges Beckie Stewart, RN, and Ronald Gordon, BS, RRT, for reviewing this chapter and for their suggestions. The author also thanks Karen McMasters for her secretarial assistance.

## References

1. Bancalari E: Bronchopulmonary dysplasia, Journal of the Florida Medical Association 70, 1983, pp. 802–807.
2. Rosenfield W: Ventilatory management: Strategies in weaning (Chapter 23) *in* Bancalari E, and Stocker JT, eds.: Bronchopulmonary Dysplasia, Washington, Hemisphere Publishing Corporation, 1988, pp. 366–369.
3. Morray J, et al.: Clinical correlates of successful weaning from mechanical ventilation in severe bronchopulmonary dysplasia, Critical Care Medicine 9(12), 1981, pp. 815–818.
4. Cloherty J, and Stark A, eds.: Manual of Neonatal Care, 2nd ed., Boston/Toronto, 1985, Little, Brown, pp. 200–202.
5. Thibeault D, and Gregory G: Neonatal Pulmonary Care, Menlo Park, California, 1979, Addison-Wesley, pp. 410–419.
6. Gerhardt T, et al.: Serial lung function measurements in infants with chronic lung disease (abstract), Pediatric Research 17, 1983, p. 376A.
7. O'Brodovich H, and Mellins R: State of the art—bronchopulmonary dysplasia, unresolved neonatal acute lung injury, American Review of Respiratory Diseases 132, 1985, pp. 694–709.
8. Nielson L: Pulmonary oxygen toxicity and other hazards of oxygen therapy, American Journal of Nursing 80(12), 1980, p. 2213.
9. Melnick G, et al.: Normal pulmonary vascular resistance and left ventricular hypertrophy in young infants with bronchopulmonary dysplasia: Echocardiographic and pathologic study, Pediatrics 66, 1980, pp. 589–596.
10. Halliday H, Dumpit F, and Brady J: Effects of inspired oxygen on echocardiographic assessment of pulmonary vascular resistance and myocardial contractility in bronchopulmonary dysplasia, Pediatrics 65, 1980, pp. 536–540.
11. Abman S, et al.: Pulmonary vascular response to oxygen in infants with severe bronchopulmonary dysplasia, Pediatrics 75, 1985, pp. 80–84.
12. Mcfadden R: Decreasing respiratory compromise during infant suctioning, American Journal of Nursing 81(12), 1981, p. 2158.

13. Voyles I: Bronchopulmonary dysplasia, American Journal of Nursing 81(3), 1981, pp. 510–511.
14. Teague W, Heldt G, and Tooley W: Hypoxia causes bronchoconstriction in infants with chronic lung disease (abstract), Pediatric Research 20, 1986, p. 443A.
15. Fox W, Scharty I, and Shaffer T: Pulmonary physiotherapy in neonates: Physiologic changes and respiratory management, Journal of Pediatrics 92, 1978, pp. 977–981.
16. Peabody J, et al.: Transcutaneous oxygen tension in sick infants, American Review of Respiratory Disease 118, 1978, pp. 83–87.
17. Rome E, et al.: Limitations of transcutaneous $PO_2$ and $PCO_2$ monitoring in infants with bronchopulmonary dysplasia, Pediatrics 74, 1984, pp. 217–220.
18. Hamilton P, Whitehead M, and Reynolds E: Underestimation of arterial oxygen tension by transcutaneous electrode with increasing age in infants, Archives of Disease in Children 60, 1985, pp. 1162–1165.
19. Satish M, and Douglas K: Transcutaneous oxygen monitoring ($TcPO_2$) (abstract), Pediatric Research 20, 1986, p. 360A.
20. Ramanathan R, Durand M, and Larrazabel C: Pulse oximetry in very low birthweight infants with acute and chronic lung disease, Pediatrics 79(4), April 1987, pp. 612–617.
21. Solimano A, et al.: Pulse oximetry advantages in infants with bronchopulmonary dysplasia, Pediatrics 78(5), November 1986, pp. 844–849.
22. Barnes C, Asonye U, and Vidyasagar D: The effects of bronchopulmonary hygiene on $P_{tC}O_2$ values in critically ill neonates, Critical Care Medicine 9(12), 1981, pp. 819–822.
23. Avery ME, and Taeusch HW, eds.: Schaffer's Diseases of the Newborn, 5th ed., Philadelphia, 1984, W.B. Saunders, p. 149.
24. Fanaroff A, and Martin R, eds.: Behrman's Neonatal-Perinatal Medicine, 3rd ed., St. Louis/Toronto, 1983, C.V. Mosby, pp. 474–475.
25. Garg M, et al.: Clinically unsuspected hypoxia during sleep and feeding in infants with bronchopulmonary dysplasia, Pediatrics 81(5), May 1988, pp. 635–642.
26. Reid L: Bronchopulmonary dysplasia—pathology, Journal of Pediatrics 95, 1979, pp. 836–841.
27. Miller R, et al.: Tracheobronchial abnormalities in infants with bronchopulmonary dysplasia, Journal of Pediatrics 111(5), November 1987, pp. 779–782.
28. Etches P, and Scott B: Chest physiotherapy in the newborn: Effect on secretions removed, Pediatrics 62, 1978, pp. 713–715.
29. Edwards D: Radiographic aspects of BPD, Journal of Pediatrics 95, 1979, pp. 823–828.
30. Bancalari E: Management of respiratory failure in the newborn, part 2, Lessons and Current Reviews in Respiratory Therapy vol. 2, 1979, pp. 75–79.
31. Kao L, et al.: Comparison of drug therapy in infants with BPD (abstract), Pediatric Research 20, 1986, p. 351A.
32. Kao L, et al.: Furosemide acutely decreases airway resistance in chronic bronchopulmonary dysplasia, Journal of Pediatrics 103, 1983, pp. 624–628.
33. Green R: The use of diuretics in infants with the respiratory distress syndrome, Seminars in Perinatology 6, 1982, pp. 172–177.
34. Brackbill Y, Douthitt T, and West H: Psychophysiologic effects in the neonate of prone versus supine placement, Journal of Pediatrics 82(1), 1973, pp. 82–84.

35. Lioy J, and Manginello F: A comparison of prone and supine positioning in the immediate post extubation period of neonates, Journal of Pediatrics 112(6), June 1988, pp. 982–984.

36. Martin R, et al.: Effects of supine and prone positions on arterial oxygen tension in the preterm infant, Pediatrics 63(4), 1979, pp. 528–531.

37. Hagaman M, et al.: Improved oxygenation and lung compliance with prone positioning of neonates, Journal of Pediatrics 94(5), May 1979, pp. 789–791.

38. Nickerson B: BPD, chronic pulmonary disease following neonatal respiratory failure, Chest 87, April 1985, pp. 528–535.

CHAPTER 3

# Complications in Infants with Bronchopulmonary Dysplasia

*Rosalyn Feller Scherf, RNC*
*NorthShore Medical Center*
*Miami, Florida*
*Susan Arndt Park, RN, BSN*
*Harborview General Hospital*
*Seattle, Washington*

Infants with bronchopulmonary dysplasia (BPD) develop multisystem complications. Depending on the severity of BPD, the complications can be minimal and limited or severe and devastating. The disease is complicated primarily by respiratory problems, which directly or indirectly affect other systems. In addition, treatments for one problem may lead to undesirable effects and complications in another system. Complications of various organ systems are listed in Table 1.

## Respiratory Complications

### Pulmonary Hypertension

In infants with BPD, pulmonary hypertension is a profound complication with far-reaching effects. If it persists, right-sided heart failure with cardiomegaly, hepatomegaly, and fluid retention develop.[1]

The combination of parenchymal lung disease seen in BPD and chronic hypoxemia can lead to pulmonary hypertension in the following way: hypoxemia leads to metabolic acidemia and together they cause pulmonary vasoconstriction. The pulmonary pressure then rises above aortic pressure result-

**TABLE 1 ■ Complications in Infants with BPD**

| RESPIRATORY | CARDIOVASCULAR SYSTEM | CENTRAL NERVOUS SYSTEM |
|---|---|---|
| Atelectasis<br>Pulmonary edema<br>Pulmonary hypertension<br>Bronchospasm<br>Lower respiratory infections<br>Bronchitis or bronchiolitis | Patent ductus arteriosus<br>Cor pulmonale<br>Systemic systolic hypertension | Cerebral palsy<br>Mental retardation<br>Blindness<br>Deafness |
| **GASTROINTESTINAL SYSTEM** | **MUSCULOSKELETAL SYSTEM** | **MISCELLANEOUS** |
| Failure to sustain normal growth & development<br>Inguinal hernia<br>Hepatic damage<br>Gastrointestinal reflux | Rickets | Electrolyte imbalance<br>Fluid retention & edema<br>Middle ear disease<br>Midline palatal defects<br>Possible increased incidence of SIDS<br>Nephrolithiasis<br>Cholelithiasis<br>Developmental and social abnormalities<br>Financial stress for families |

ing in decreased pulmonary blood flow and increased pulmonary vascular resistance. The decrease in pulmonary blood flow also diminishes the amount of oxygenated blood from the pulmonary vessels that returns to the heart, thereby worsening the hypoxemia.

BPD also leads to an increase in intrapleural pressure due to hyperexpansion of the lungs. This can interfere with venous return to the right heart, which increases pulmonary vascular resistance. The resulting pulmonary vasoconstriction can increase right-to-left shunting through the foramen ovale or ductus arteriosus, which in turn increases hypoxemia. Thus, the vicious cycle of lung disease and its effects on pulmonary vascular stability is established (see Figure 1).

Pulmonary hypertension resulting in cor pulmonale may account for a certain number of relatively late deaths (after six months) in children with BPD whose parenchymal lung disease may be improving. Several echocardiographic studies have shown pulmonary artery pressure to be normal as long as $PaO_2$ is maintained above 55 mmHg. Maintaining adequate tissue oxygenation will therefore possibly prevent the occurrence of pulmonary hypertension.[1]

The eagerness to discontinue supplemental oxygen can result in poor growth and the development of pulmonary hypertension.[2,3] Therefore,

**FIGURE 1 ■ Cycle of Pulmonary Hypertension in BPD**

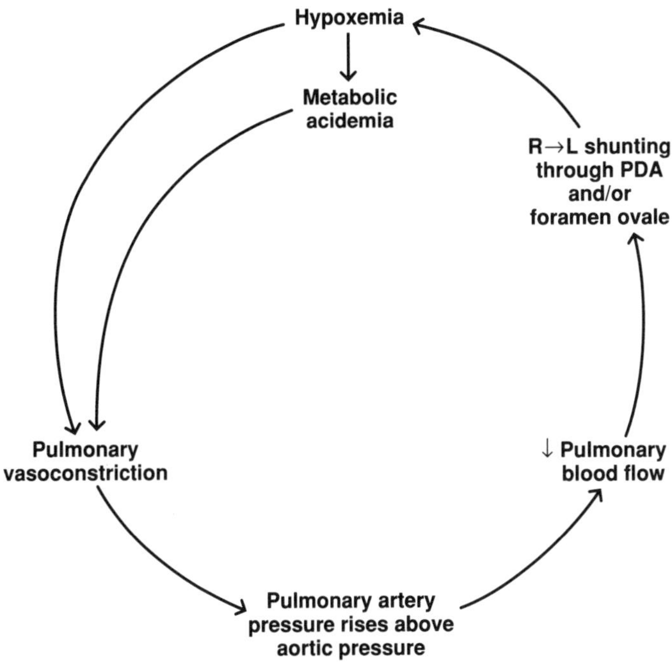


patience and appropriate consistency must be the dominant factors in weaning from supplemental oxygen.

### Atelectasis

Atelectasis is frequently seen in infants with BPD[3,4] and can cause insufficient alveolar ventilation with consequent carbon dioxide retention. The atelectasis can occur in any area of the lung but often involves the left lower lobe.[4,5] If cardiac enlargement occurs it may compress the left lower lobe bronchus, predisposing the infant to atelectasis in this area.[5] Secretions may plug the airway, resulting in collapsed alveoli. After extubation, the right upper and middle lobes are the usual sites of atelectasis. These lobes are especially vulnerable to airway collapse because they have fewer airways, and the right main bronchus is comparatively small.

Atelectasis can be prevented or improved with good pulmonary hygiene by using chest physiotherapy (CPT) and/or direct endotracheal suctioning.[2,4,5]

CPT preceding suctioning has been shown to increase the amount of secretions removed.[6,7]

### Bronchospasm

Frequently, infants with BPD will suddenly become cyanotic and have increased respiratory distress when they are handled or when crying or fussing. Sometimes this is accompanied by bradycardia. The infant becomes difficult to ventilate whether he is on a ventilator or being hand ventilated with high inspiratory pressures. Wheezing is commonly present during these episodes. The pathophysiology of these episodes and the optimal treatment for them are not well known.[3] The occurrence of bronchospasm could, however, be secondary to severe irritation of the airways, especially during ventilation or in the presence of a respiratory infection.

Nevertheless, it is known that these infants have hypertrophy of peribronchiolar smooth muscle, increased airway resistance, hyperactive airways, and a decrease in compliance.[1,2,7,8] Their chest x-rays usually show areas of hyperinflation. Some investigators have found aerosol bronchodilators to be effective in improving lung function by decreasing airway resistance and increasing lung compliance.[2,9-11] The bronchodilators relax the smooth muscle and therefore alleviate the airway obstruction. Therefore, a trial of bronchodilators in infants having these episodes of bronchospasm may be beneficial, resulting ultimately in improved oxygenation and ventilation. (See Chapter 4 for information on the use of bronchodilators.)

### Pulmonary Edema

Pulmonary edema refers to excessive fluid in the alveoli or pulmonary interstitial spaces. There is concern that pulmonary edema, caused by an increase in pulmonary blood flow and an increase in interstitial lung fluid, contributes to the development of BPD in the preterm infant.[1,2] Factors that influence the occurrence of pulmonary edema in the preterm infant include excessive fluid intake and the presence of a patent ductus arteriosus with left-to-right shunting.[7] The higher degree of ventilatory support necessary to ventilate a lung with increased fluid content may produce worsening lung disease as well.[1]

In a healthy infant, water and solutes are moving continuously out of the vascular space. The solutes enter the interstitium of the lung and are cleared by the lymphatics. Perhaps they are also cleared by the venular end of the microcirculation.[12] Infants with BPD appear to have a predisposition to fluid accumulation in the lung. They may even handle a normal fluid intake poorly.

It is still not known why this occurs.[1] It is felt that this fluid accumulation is due to alterations in the following:

1. Pulmonary vascular resistance. Hypoxia and in some cases left ventricular dysfunction may result in an increase in pulmonary vascular pressure.[2,4] Perhaps this is why clinical improvement is observed when early treatment of hypoxia is initiated in infants with a PDA.
2. Plasma oncotic pressure. Total protein concentrations have been shown to be lower in infants of younger gestational age.[4] Decreased plasma concentration in addition to poor nutrition may be the cause of the change in plasma oncotic pressure.[2,5]
3. Capillary permeability. High inspired oxygen concentrations or infections of the capillary endothelium may cause increased capillary permeability in the pulmonary microvasculature.[2]

In addition, surfactant deficiency or dysfunction may increase mechanical hydrostatic forces that promote pulmonary edema.[4] Frequently, the preterm infant does not produce surfactant because of the immaturity of his enzyme system. Asphyxia, acidosis, and shock can also cause insufficient surfactant production.[4]

Lymphatic drainage may be impaired because of compression of the pulmonary lymphatics by interstitial fluid and fibrous tissue. When an infant with BPD also develops cor pulmonale, lymphatic drainage may be decreased due to increases in central venous pressure.[2] The accumulation of fluid in the lungs further compromises the infant and requires more respiratory support, which may in turn cause further damage.[2] For example, if the infant is intubated, the fluid-filled terminal conducting airways may necessitate an increase in positive end/expiratory pressure (PEEP).[4] This often intensifies the dissection of interstitial air into the pulmonary lymphatics, resulting in pneumomediastinum or extensive subpleural air. The dissection of this air may obstruct drainage of the interstitial fluid, preventing resolution of the pulmonary edema.[8]

Treatment of pulmonary edema consists of fluid and sodium restriction. If increased lung water persists, diuretic therapy can be instituted. If the infant is on a ventilator, the PEEP may be increased to decrease pulmonary blood flow. The infant's blood gases need to be followed closely to determine if the increase in PEEP is beneficial. There is currently no known approach that will return pulmonary permeability to normal.[5] (For nursing actions, see care plan in Appendix A.)

### Respiratory Infections

The first year of life for the infant with BPD is often complicated by serious respiratory infections. Infants with BPD are susceptible to a variety of upper

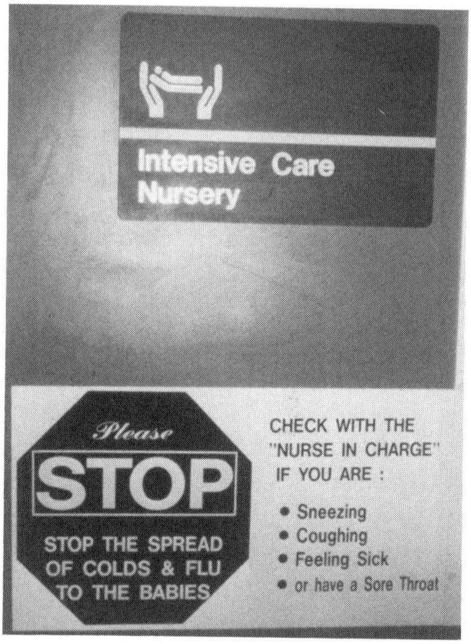


**FIGURE 2 ■ Screening both staff and visitors** for viral infections, especially during the winter months when respiratory synctial virus and adenovirus are more widespread, is an important part of prevention of upper respiratory infections in the BPD infant.

and lower respiratory infections because of their compromised respiratory status and less than optimal nutritional status. In addition, the hospitalized infant is at risk for nosocomial infections.

During the winter months respiratory syncytial virus (RSV) is frequently seen, but the influenza virus, adenovirus, parainfluenza virus and cytomegalovirus can also cause serious respiratory compromise in the BPD infant. One center reports that 59 percent of 30 BPD infants followed at home who were less than two years of age contracted RSV after discharge; consequences of the infection included lengthy rehospitalizations or stays in the intensive care unit for severe bronchiolitis or bronchopneumonia.[13] Infants most affected were those who required oxygen supplementation at the time of infection or within three months before the infection occurred. Other significant factors that determined the rate and severity of infection included age less than one year and tobacco smoke in the home.

Prevention of viral and bacterial infections is, of course, the first step. For the hospitalized infant increased surveillance of staff, visitors and others in direct contact with the BPD infant for upper respiratory infections is essential during the months of greatest incidence of viral infections, because even a mild cold in a healthy individual can seriously compromise the borderline pulmonary status of the BPD infant (Figure 2).

For the BPD infant at home, parents need to know that reducing exposure to persons with colds or other viruses and avoiding living situations with smokers are important. These infants may not be able to tolerate day care situations.

Nosocomial bacterial infections are also a concern. Thus, while the infant is still hospitalized, evaluation for sepsis is ongoing. The patient may have many potential sites for infections such as arterial lines, central venous lines, and endotracheal tubes. It is important to utilize good handwashing and sterile suctioning techniques. Equipment for oxygen therapy is also a potential reservoir for bacteria. Nebulizers are frequently colonized with gram-negative bacteria;[1] this is why many units have a standard policy of changing the complete ventilator circuit every 24 to 48 hours. Another source of bacterial infections is aspiration; feeding techniques that minimize the risk of aspiration are discussed in Chapter 5.

Early recognition of an infection can lead to prompt treatment and hopefully minimize or eliminate complications. Parents may be a good resource for their infant's baseline respiratory status, and they can provide continuity in care and observation.[14] Increases in wheezing, retractions, tachypnea, and feeding intolerances are important warning signals.[3] Bronchiolitis or bronchopneumonia are common complications following upper respiratory infections.[14]

Treatment for infections consists of increasing the frequency of suctioning and CPT. The pneumonias are usually treated with broad spectrum antibiotics, or agents such as ribavirin if RSV is documented [3,5,13] Chest x-ray examinations may aid in evaluating the status of the lungs.[3,5,14]

Infants with BPD have been shown to have a decreased pulmonary capacity. A morphometric analysis of a 33 month old infant dying from BPD showed the total number of alveoli to be 19 million, approximately 10 percent of the number of alveoli in control subjects.[15] Because the infant with BPD has so little reserve, a respiratory infection can have a great impact on his respiratory status. Bacterial or viral infections may result in acute pulmonary problems that require hospitalization (if the infant has been discharged) and in some cases may precipitate an unexpected death.[1,2,4,5] Even after the first year of life, these infants are still prone to respiratory infections.[1,3]

### Tracheobronchial Abnormalities

Tracheobronchial abnormalities are serious complications that can occur in infants with BPD who have required prolonged endotracheal intubation and assisted ventilation. A recent report reveals that 12 infants with BPD who underwent diagnostic bronchoscopy for clinical pulmonary difficulties that were unexplained by their degree of lung disease had airway abnormalities to some degree.[16] These abnormalities include tracheomalacia, granulation tissue formation at various places along the large airway, inspissated secretions, and stenosis of varying degrees. All infants studied were intubated or tracheotomized at the time of evaluation. Table 2 lists factors that can lead to laryngotracheal damage.

**TABLE 2 ■ Factors that Lead to Laryngotracheal Damage**

1. Duration of intubation
2. Duration of mechanical ventilation
3. Inadequate patient sedation
4. Repeated flexion and extension of neck
5. Patient fighting ventilator
6. Traction on tube during turning, suctioning, and ventilator connection and disconnection
7. Previous prolonged intubation
8. Chronic airway or lung disease
9. Airway infection

The premature lung and airways are vulnerable to ventilator induced damage. Presumably, the more immature the airway at the time of insult, the greater the impact on airway growth. When bronchioli and alveoli have little connective tissue support, the presence of high pressures tends to mechanically damage patent airways and parenchyma.[2] Prolonged endotracheal (ET) intubation is associated with squamous metaplasia and occasional necrosis of tracheal epithelium, resulting in disruption of normal ciliary transport of secretions from distal airways.[2,16] The humidity and temperature of inspired gas delivered by the ventilator system also greatly influence airway epithelial ciliary activity, thus contributing to tracheal damage.[17]

Frequent suctioning can also damage the epithelial membrane. Partial or complete occlusion of the trachea and even the main stem bronchi has occurred at the site of the suction catheter injury.[7] It is recommended by some authors that side-hole catheters be used, and that during suctioning catheters be advanced only as far as the distal end of the ET tube.[18]

Direct mechanical damage to underlying tracheal epithelium can be caused by ET tube pressure and friction which cause ulceration and a secondary stricture of the upper airway. Ulceration will usually heal rapidly on removal of the ET tube, but strictures can result from scar formation.

As the collagen in circumferential scar tissue contracts after extubation, tracheal stenosis may progress over a period of weeks, resulting in obliteration of the airway lumen.[3] Damage to the subglottic area produces varying degrees of stenosis. A prospective study of a hundred infants intubated over seven days reported a total incidence of subglottic stenosis of 10 percent; six infants had moderate stenosis and four had severe stenosis. The mean birthweight of the study infants was 1309 gms, and the mean gestational age was 29.5 weeks. Factors that correlated with the development of stenosis were duration of intubation, days of mechanical ventilation, number of times intubated and presence of post-extubation stridor.[19]

The signs of stenosis in milder forms may not appear immediately after extubation, but may occur later in the first year of life when the infant has a superimposed respiratory tract infection. During discharge planning and instruction, parents should be informed of the possibility of airway obstruction in their infant during respiratory infections. They should be familiar with the signs of upper airway obstruction and told to seek medical assistance immediately if the infant develops stridor or any other signs of upper airway distress. If obstruction is severe, a tracheostomy may be necessary. Once a tracheostomy is performed, parents must be thoroughly instructed in proper tracheostomy care.

## Cardiovascular Complications

### Patent Ductus Arteriosus

The role of the patent ductus arteriosus (PDA) is felt to be an important factor in the development of BPD.[1,3] Not all infants with BPD, however, are diagnosed with a clinically significant PDA. Nevertheless, a high percentage of these infants have this left to right shunt.[3,7,20] Pulmonary congestion is caused from the excessive blood flow through this shunt. This in turn causes the blood to shunt increasingly left to right,[3] and a vicious cycle develops. $FiO_2$ and ventilator settings usually need to be raised as a result of the physiological changes from the PDA, resulting in more barotrauma and oxygen toxicity to pulmonary tissue. Additional pulmonary damage may be caused by the increased blood flow.[3]

Early detection of a PDA can have a significant impact on the treatment of patients with BPD. The following are some of the early warning signals:

1. A frequently heard systolic murmur. However, not all PDAs have audible murmurs.[2,3]
2. An increase in cardiac size. This may be difficult to visualize on x-ray because of pulmonary infiltrates and atelectasis.[3]
3. Decreased diastolic blood pressure, bounding pulses, hepatomegaly, excessive weight gain, pulmonary edema, rales, and increased respiratory rate.[2,3]
4. Increased blood flow through the left atrium, causing it to become dilated.

All these problems can be further aggravated by excessive fluid intake. Echocardiograms are usually ordered to confirm the diagnosis of a PDA.

Medical management is frequently the first method of choice in the attempt to close the PDA. Fluid overload is treated by fluid restriction and/or the administration of diuretics.[3,21,22] The prostaglandin inhibitor, indomethacin, can also be used in an attempt to medically close the PDA. If medical management is unsuccessful, surgical intervention may be necessary.[3]

When the ductus is closed or decreases in size, it is frequently possible to begin lowering oxygen and/or ventilator settings. It is important to note, however, that stress and/or a hypoxic insult can cause the PDA to reopen if it has not been surgically ligated.

## Cor Pulmonale

Cor pulmonale is a cardiovascular complication resulting from chronic pulmonary hypertension. Pulmonary hypertension causes an increased workload for the right side of the heart. This in turn causes pulmonary edema and right ventricular hypertrophy. The right ventricular hypertrophy progresses to right-sided heart failure with right ventricular dilatation, cardiomegaly, hepatomegaly and peripheral edema.[22]

Right ventricular failure and subsequent cor pulmonale are seen less frequently today,[1] probably as a result of maintaining $PaO_2$ at higher levels (>55 mm Hg). In addition, careful monitoring to eliminate hypoxic swings and more conservative respiratory management when weaning from supplemental oxygen have contributed to the reduction in this complication for BPD infants.

In some patients cor pulmonale still can occur despite careful monitoring due to an extremely labile respiratory course. A hospital course punctuated by repeated bronchospasms, bacterial or viral infection or other complications can result in hypoxia-induced chronic pulmonary hypertension that eventually leads to cor pulmonale. Early identification of cor pulmonale is important, as it can be life threatening.

When caring for infants with cor pulmonale, the following factors are considered:

- Often the infant will be on fluid restrictions to prevent further fluid overload and/or will be given diuretics.[3]
- The infant needs to be monitored for dehydration as well as fluid overload.
- Potassium supplements may need to be given if the infant is on diuretics.
- The number of calories the child will receive may be limited because of the fluid restriction.
- Digitalis may be given to increase cardiac output. (For further nursing actions see the care plan in Appendix B.)

## Systemic Hypertension

Systemic hypertension has been reported as a significant complication in BPD infants. In one report, 43 percent of a group of 30 infants developed systemic hypertension (defined as a systolic pressure >113 mm Hg on three occasions) during the first year of life. Although the hypertension was either transient or easily controlled with antihypertensive medication, several infants showed cardiac effects from hypertension (left ventricular hypertrophy) and one infant suffered a cerebral vascular accident as a consequence. The cause of the systemic hypertension in these patients was not obvious; however, the authors speculate that perhaps chronic intermittent hypoxia may have been a factor.[23]

Systemic hypertension can also be caused by some of the pharmacologic agents used to treat BPD, such as steroids. Hypertension can also potentially result from renal calcifications, a complication of chronic diuretic therapy. Thus, careful monitoring of blood pressure in BPD infants during hospitalization and in follow-up is essential, and appropriate treatment of hypertension is an important aspect of care.

## Gastrointestinal and Nutritional Complications

### Failure to Sustain Normal Growth and Development

Nutrition plays a dominant role in the recovery process of infants with BPD. These infants' specific nutritional needs are not fully known, but they normally have excessive energy (calorie) requirements. Follow-up studies have shown that although head circumference is normal, these infants are below the third percentile for height and weight even at five years of age.[1,24] In addition, calories are necessary to aid in repair of lung tissue. Without a positive nitrogen balance, lung tissue cannot grow. Inadequate nutrition delays somatic growth, the development of new alveoli, and the enlargement of the airway diameter.[25]

Maintaining adequate nutrition in these infants is frequently difficult because their caloric requirements are greater than those for infants who do not have BPD.[1,26] Some of these infants require up to 180 calories/kg/day to achieve adequate weight gain. In infants receiving theophylline, metabolic rate may be increased, further increasing caloric needs.

The infants' work of breathing is several-fold that of normal preterm or full-term infants. Because of this, many of these infants may have a 25 percent increase in their resting oxygen consumption, thereby increasing their caloric requirements.[27] Oxygen consumption is also increased during feedings. Infants with BPD are more vulnerable to respiratory muscle fatigue. They may tire easily during feedings, fail to suck adequate volumes, and thus need to be gavage fed. Nasogastric or oral tube feeding, unless more stressful in the older infants, should be given until a steady weight gain is noted and respirations are easier and less labored. If the infant is kept NPO during an acute phase of illness, as with sepsis, total parenteral nutrition is recommended if he is unable to resume feedings. This is essential to maintaining an adequate caloric intake.

Sufficient oxygenation improves the rate of weight gain.[7] Thus, maintaining an adequate $PaO_2$ is essential. Appropriate weight gain increases chest wall strength, improves pulmonary mechanics, and decreases the work of breathing.[1,25] This, in turn, makes more calories available for somatic growth and additional adequate weight gain, which is the ultimate nutritional goal. The role of nutrition in BPD is discussed in Chapter 5.

**FIGURE 3 ■ X–ray of a five month old infant with stage IV BPD and multiple healing rib fractures (see arrows).** This infant's course was complicated by severe osteopenia due to prolonged parenteral nutrition and diuretic therapy.

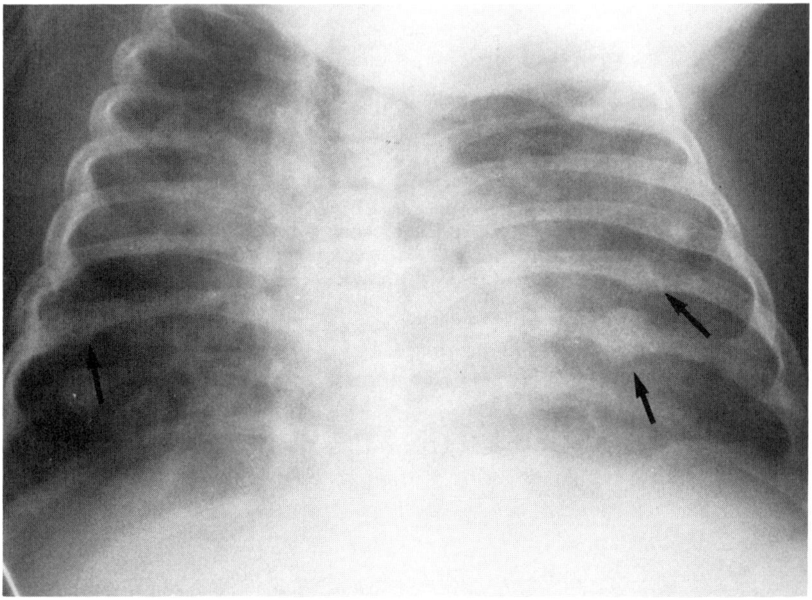

## Rickets

Rickets may be found in infants with BPD; the cause is multifactorial.[3,5,7,24] The majority of the deposition of calcium into the bones occurs during the last two months of gestation. Because most infants who develop BPD are born prematurely, this deposition of calcium is deficient. In addition, because of the difficulty in meeting the nutritional needs of these infants, dietary and/or parenteral alimentation intake of calcium, phosphorous, and vitamin D may also be deficient.

Calcium losses in urine output during chronic furosemide administration compound the situation. With adequate exposure to sunlight, there is no dietary requirement for vitamin D. These infants are rarely, however, outdoors in the sunlight and therefore lack this means of vitamin D supplementation.

The alteration in calcium and phosphate homeostasis has undesirable effects on bone growth. Fractures may readily occur. Because many of these infants receive CPT to loosen pulmonary secretions, they are particularly susceptible to rib fractures.[5,6] The rib fractures are usually diagnosed on routine chest x-ray examinations (see Figure 3). If rib fractures are discovered, x-ray examinations should be done to evaluate wrists and knees. The metaphyses of knees and wrists are particularly sensitive indicators of rickets. X-rays will show metaphyseal fraying, widening, and cupping occuring in true cases of rickets.[5]

In the presence of vitamin D deficiency, these infants will show a decrease in the concentration of inorganic phosphorous and an increase in alkaline phosphatase.

All infants with BPD should be observed closely for any signs of fractures:

1. Abnormal protrusions of bone
2. Palpation of round, bony masses (the round callus formation that occurs during the healing process)
3. Swelling of joints or other areas
4. Excessive crying (as if in pain) when moving extremities or during CPT
5. One limb shorter than the other
6. An unnatural movement in a normally rigid area

Treatment usually consists of giving vitamin D, 400 IU daily, treating fractures (by immobilizing a leg or shoulder, for example), discontinuing CPT, and providing more calcium. If absolutely necessary, CPT may be continued very cautiously.

## Inguinal Hernia

Infants with BPD have a high incidence of inguinal hernias.[3] In general, these hernias occur more frequently in boys, especially on the right side, but bilateral inguinal hernias are not uncommon.[27] The hernia is usually diagnosed when a mass is detected in the inguinal region or in the scrotum. Initially, it usually is noticeable when the infant is crying or straining and less noticeable when he is sleeping or inactive. At a later stage, it may remain constantly visible and palpable. Many of these infants may be uncommonly irritable and cry frequently, as though in pain, for several weeks before the hernia is apparent.[28]

Surgery is recommended as soon as possible because there is a risk of incarceration and strangulation of the hernia. However, anesthesia for infants with BPD poses a risk. Elective surgery should be carefully planned. If possible, surgery should be delayed until the infant is in optimum medical condition. In the interim, measures to reduce the hernia are performed. If unable to reduce the hernia, surgery is necessary immediately to prevent strangulation. Prior to surgery, the anesthesiologist should be fully informed of the infant's present respiratory status as well as additional medical problems. Optimal postoperative care with particular attention to monitoring and evaluating of respiratory function is essential.

## Developmental and Social Complications

These two areas are very complex and are briefly discussed here. They are elaborated in Chapters 6 and 7.

A report in the late 1970s concluded that 34 percent of the infants with BPD had one or more of the following problems: cerebral palsy, mental retardation, deafness, and blindness.[29] Other studies reported similar findings.[30,31] Nevertheless, compared with a group of infants with severe hyaline membrane disease but without BPD who were ventilated more than 24 hours, there was no significant difference in the degree of handicap.[29] The CNS complications might be due to the hypoxic insults to the brain occurring during the periods of respiratory distress and associated problems rather than the ventilation itself.[31] The extent and degree of injury depends upon the maturity of the brain tissue at the time of the insult. Therefore, infants born prior to 32–34 weeks gestation are more vulnerable.

A recent report discusses another neurologic finding: a progressive neurologic disorder that occurs later during the disease and is unrelated to earlier CNS insults such as IVH and asphyxia. In this disorder, infants as old as three months of age began to exhibit neurologic deterioration, unexplained intermittent fevers with convulsions, and a leveling off of head growth in spite of appropriate weight gain. Of the five patients with this disorder described in the article, all eventually died. Etiology is unknown, but it seems to be related to the course and treatment of severe BPD.[32]

In regards to the development of varying degrees of blindness, which is due to retinopathy of prematurity, the effect of oxygen on retinal vessels depends on (1) the stage of development of the retinal vessels, (2) the length of exposure to oxygen, and (3) the partial pressure of oxygen in arterial blood.[33] The development of hearing impairments is multifactorial, including hypoxia, ototoxic medications, CNS infections, and excessive noise. These risk factors are compounded by the increased incidence of otitis media in this population.

Infants with BPD also experience a lack of normal sensory stimulation and social interaction. They are isolated from the normal social environment by their oxygen and ventilatory requirements. Their irritability and sudden episodes of cyanosis and/or bradycardia frequently frighten those who are caring for them. Medical personnel, parents, and even nursing personnel sometimes find it very difficult to handle and interact with these infants because of these episodes. Therefore, at times, the amount of stimuli normally given to infants of comparable age is limited for infants with BPD.

These infants are repeatedly exposed to unavoidable painful or uncomfortable stimuli (for example, blood being drawn). Their oxygen and/or ventilator apparatus and IVs in some cases limit their ability to practice such gross motor skills as rolling over and sitting up.

There is interference in the maternal-infant bonding process as well as in the bonding process with the father. If there are siblings, the family unit can be disrupted even further because of the uncertainty of the infant's outcome as well as the adjustment to a new and potentially handicapped brother or sister. Some parents may feel frightened and inadequate; others are angry and hostile.

Mothers and fathers of infants with BPD must deal with multiple adjustments, frustrations, and emotional burdens that can be overwhelming. Frequently, fathers feel they must assume the role of being the "strong," "sturdy" head of the family who must remain calm and composed. However, these fathers also have to deal with some deep and conflicting emotions during a time in which they feel they are required to be supportive and strong. Not only is bonding with his child interrupted, but feelings of guilt and anger may adversely affect his relationship with his wife.

These feelings can occur when parents need each other's support, acceptance, and understanding the most. Both parents may lose valuable time from work or may have to go to work when they would rather be with their infant. This can also intensify concerns about financial responsibilities. The financial burdens that parents incur as a result of this disease can be overwhelming and devastating. Hospital bills can be staggering.

The emotional deprivation these infants experience because of the severity of their illness, along with chronic hypoxia, suboptimal growth patterns, and prolonged hospitalization, compound the problems of psychosocial development.

The following interventions can help lessen the impact of these complications:

1. Provide adequate psychosensory stimulation for the infant whenever possible and appropriate.
2. Reduce the number of painful or unpleasant stimuli.
3. Help the parents to feel their infant belongs to them and help them to care for their infant. Their observations can provide continuity of care. Their reports to the health care team of changes in the infant's behavior patterns or responses can be valuable in detecting early warning signals of impending complications.
4. Allow the parents to have some control over their infant's social and sensory development.
5. Provide adequate information for the parents in regards to available financial assistance, social services, parent support groups, and discharge planning.

One last area of concern is that of mortality. The rate of mortality in infants with BPD is between 30 and 40 percent.[20,29] This has been noticeably reduced since the disease was first described by Northway and associates.[1] Overall improvement in the care of these infants has probably contributed to the decrease in mortality. Those who do succumb usually do so because of progressive pulmonary disease, sepsis, and/or intractable cor pulmonale.[1,21,29]

Westhammer and associates report that 11 percent of infants with BPD who were discharged from the hospital later died with a postmortem diagnosis of SIDS.[34] In general, infants with BPD are at risk to die unexpectedly.[1] Therefore, parents should be given training in CPR and provided with ample discharge planning and follow-up resources; cardiorespiratory monitoring may also be indicated.

Although there are infants with developmental complications, there is also a large number of surviving infants who do not have these complications and who, at present, appear to be developing normally.[31]

### Miscellaneous Complications

Other complications can develop in infants with BPD, including the following:

1. Electrolyte imbalance, especially when potent diuretics are used[1] (Some of the problems include hyponatremia, hypercalciuria, metabolic alkalosis, hypokalemia, and hypochloremia. Hypochloremia, when due to the use of diuretics, will promote bicarbonate retention, an undesirable effect in chronic hypercarbia.)
2. Fluid retention and edema
3. Cholestatic jaundice (from prolonged hyperalimentation)
4. A high incidence of otitis media
5. Bronchitis or bronchiolitis, which is common during the first one to two years of life
6. Gastroesophageal reflux (This frequently occurs in infants with BPD but its exact significance is still disputed.[35] See Chapter 5 for more information.)
7. Nephrolithiasis, due to diuretic therapy and increased urinary calcium excretion[36,37]
8. Cholelithiasis, due to furosemide therapy[38,39]
9. Intractable respiratory failure
10. Overwhelming sepsis, which can be terminal

The main nursing, respiratory, and medical goals should aim toward preventing these complications. If complications do arise, we should seek to minimize their effects. A shift in focus from immediate recovery to a more realistic, patient approach is highly recommended: These infants have a chronic illness that takes time to resolve.

Astute observations of these infants, with early and prompt detection of warning signals, can lead to appropriate and timely interventions. Early interventions can decrease the severity of complications, possibly interrupting the vicious cycle of problems. This in turn can potentially decrease morbidity and length of hospitalization and improve the infant's outcome. In addition, the social and financial complications for both patients and their families may be diminished.

## Acknowledgment

The authors gratefully acknowledge Constance M. O'Hara, RN, BSN, and Charles Torrence, RN, for reviewing this chapter and for their suggestions. The authors also thank Jo Ann Jarrett for her secretarial assistance.

## References

1. Bancalari E, and Gerhardt T: Bronchopulmonary dysplasia, Pediatric Clinics of North America 33(1), February 1986, pp. 1–20.
2. O'Brodovich H, and Mellins R: State of the art—bronchopulmonary dysplasia, unresolved neonatal acute lung injury, American Review of Respiratory Diseases, July-December 1985, pp. 694–709.
3. Nickerson B: BPD, chronic pulmonary disease following neonatal respiratory failure, Chest 87, April 1985, pp. 528–535.
4. Goldberg R, and Bancalari E: Bronchopulmonary dysplasia: Clinical presentation and the role of mechanical ventilation, Respiratory Care 31(7), July 1986, pp. 591–596.
5. Edwards D: Radiographic aspects of bronchopulmonary dysplasia, Journal of Pediatrics 95, 1979, pp. 823–828.
6. Etches P, and Scott B: Chest physiotherapy in the newborn: Effect on secretions removed, Pediatrics 62, 1978, pp. 713–715.
7. Fanaroff A, and Martin R, eds.: Behrman's Neonatal-Perinatal Medicine, 3rd ed., St. Louis, 1983, C.V. Mosby, pp. 439, 469–475.
8. Melnick G, et al.: Normal pulmonary vascular resistance and left ventricular hypertrophy in young infants with bronchopulmonary dysplasia: Echocardiographic and pathologic study, Pediatrics 66, 1980, pp. 589–596.
9. Fox W, Scharty I, and Shaffer T: Pulmonary physiotherapy in neonates: Physiologic changes and respiratory management, Journal of Pediatrics 92, 1978, pp. 977–981.
10. Kao L, et al.: Comparison of drug therapy in infants with BPD (abstract), Pediatric Research 20, 1986, p. 315A.
11. Karp T, and Harris T: Neonatal bronchospasm and its complications, Perinatology/Neonatology, June 1985, pp. 35–37.
12. O'Brodovich H: Pulmonary edema in unresolved neonatal acute lung injury, bronchopulmonary dysplasia in related chronic respiratory disorders, Report of the Ninetieth Ross Conference on Pediatric Research, March 1986, pp. 69–74.

13. Groothius J, Gutierrez K, and Lauer B: Respiratory syncytial virus infection in children with bronchopulmonary dysplasia, Pediatrics 82(2), August 1988, pp. 199–203.

14. Koops B, Abman S, and Accarso F: Outpatient management and follow-up of bronchopulmonary dysplasia, Clinics in Perinatology 11(1), February 1984, pp. 101–122.

15. Sobonya R, et al.: Morphometric analysis of the lung in prolonged bronchopulmonary dysplasia, Pediatric Research 16, 1982, pp. 969–972.

16. Miller R, et al.: Tracheobronchial abnormalities in infants with bronchopulmonary dysplasia, Journal of Pediatrics 3(5), November 1987, pp. 779–782.

17. Ehrenkranz R, Ablow R, and Warshaw J: Oxygen toxicity: The complication of oxygen use in the newborn infant, Clinics in Perinatology 5, 1978, pp. 442–443.

18. Bailey C, et al.: Shallow versus deep endotracheal suctioning in young rabbits: pathologic effects on the tracheobronchial wall, Pediatrics 82(5), November 1988, pp. 746–751.

19. Sherman J, et al.: Factors influencing acquired subglottic stenosis in infants, Journal of Pediatrics 109(2), August 1986, pp. 322–327.

20. Korones S, and Lancaster J: High-Risk Newborn Infants: The Basis for Intensive Care, 3rd ed., St. Louis, 1981, C.V. Mosby, pp. 221–227.

21. Bancalari E, et al.: BPD: Clinical presentation, Journal of Pediatrics 95, 1979, pp. 819–823.

22. Hirschfeld S: Cor pulmonale: Diagnosis and significance, Journal of the Florida Medical Association 70, 1983, pp. 59–66.

23. Abman S, et al.: Systemic hypertension in infants with bronchopulmonary dysplasia, Journal of Pediatrics, June 1984, pp. 928–931.

24. Farrell P, ed.: Nutrition and infant lung functions: Report of a national heart, lung, and blood institute symposium, Pediatric Pulmonology 2(1), January-February 1986, pp. 44–59.

25. Gerhardt T, et al.: Serial lung function measurements in infants with chronic lung disease (abstract), Pediatric Research 17, 1983, p. 376A.

26. Stahlmann M: Clinical description of BPD, Journal of Pediatrics 95, 1979, pp. 829–834.

27. Weinstein M, and Oh W: Oxygen consumption in infants with bronchopulmonary dysplasia, Journal of Pediatrics 99, 1981, pp. 958–961.

28. Avery ME, and Taeusch HW, eds.: Schaffer's Diseases of the Newborn 5th ed., Philidelphia, 1984, W.B. Saunders, p. 360.

29. Northway W: Observations on BPD, Journal of Pediatrics 95, 1979, pp. 815–817.

30. Yu V, et al.: Growth and development of very low birthweight infants recovering from bronchopulmonary dysplasia, Archives of Diseases in Childhood 58, 1983, pp. 791–794.

31. Fitzhardinge P: Follow-up studies in infants treated by mechanical ventilation, Clinics in Perinatology 5, 1978, pp. 451–456.

32. Campbell L, McAlister W, and Volpe J: Neurologic aspects of bronchopulmonary dysplasia, Clinical Pediatrics 27(1), January 1988, pp. 7–13.

33. Lucey JF, and Dangman B: A reexamination of the role of oxygen in RLF, Pediatrics 73, 1984, pp. 82–96.

34. Westhammer J, et al.: Sudden infant death syndrome in infants with bronchopulmonary dysplasia, Pediatrics 69, 1982, pp. 301–304.

35. Hoyoux C, et al.: Chronic bronchopulmonary disease and gastroesophageal reflux in children, Pediatric Pulmonology 1(3), May/June 1985, pp. 149–153.

36. Gilsanz V, et al.: Nephrolithiasis in premature infants, Radiology 154, 1985, pp. 107–110.

37. Hufnagle K, et al.: Renal calcifications: A complication of long term furosemide therapy in premature infants, Pediatrics 70, 1982, pp. 360–363.

38. Bunjapen C, Howell C, and Kanto W: Cholecystitis in a premature infant, Clinical Pediatrics 25, 1986, pp. 96–97.

39. Brill P, Winchester P, and Rosen M: Neonatal cholelithiasis, Pediatric Radiology 12, 1982, pp. 285–288.

## CHAPTER 4

# Pharmacologic Treatment of Bronchopulmonary Dysplasia

*David J. Durand, MD, FAAP*
*Children's Hospital*
*Oakland, California*

*Lily C. Kao, MD, FAAP*
*Children's Hospital*
*Oakland, California*

There is no cure for bronchopulmonary dysplasia (BPD). Our role must be to support these patients while they outgrow the disease by gradually growing new, healthier lung tissue. Thus, all of our efforts should be directed toward maximizing growth and minimizing iatrogenic complications. This includes meticulous attention to the details of nutrition, ventilation, oxygen supplementation, treatment of intercurrent infections, and psychosocial support of both the infant and the family. In addition to these modalities, we must also do what we can to optimize the pulmonary function of the infant with BPD. Pharmacologic intervention is the key to improving pulmonary function.

After a brief review of the role of the pulmonary function test (PFT) in evaluating pulmonary status in infants with BPD, we discuss the use of diuretics, bronchodilators, and other more experimental agents in the treatment of these infants.

For the past five years, we have systematically studied the pulmonary function abnormalities of infants with BPD and their optimal pharmacologic treatment. We have performed more than 200 PFTs in infants with BPD,

**TABLE 1 ■ Common Pulmonary Function Tests (PFT), What They Measure, and the Usual Abnormalities in Infants with BPD**

| PFT (Abbreviation) | Measures | Abnormality in BPD |
|---|---|---|
| Dynamic pulmonary compliance (Cdyn) | Lung "stiffness" | Decreased because of pulmonary edema and fibrosis |
| Airway resistance (Raw) | Obstruction of large, medium airways | Increased because of abnormal airway structure and bronchospasm |
| Maximal expiratory flow at FRC (VmaxFRC) | Obstruction of small airways | Increased for same reason as Raw |
| Thoracic gas volume (TGV) | Amount of air remaining in lung after exhalation | Increased because of air trapping |
| Functional residual capacity (FRC) | Same as TGV | Same as TGV |

Other PFTs used in some studies: Respiratory system compliance (Crs), Respiratory system resistance (Rrs), Specific airway conductance (SGaw)

without encountering complications. We have shown that these tests are accurate, reproducible, and a good indicator of severity of pulmonary disease in infants with BPD.[1]

Pulmonary function tests are closer to the "gold standard" for evaluating the pulmonary status of infants with BPD than other techniques such as physical examination, blood gas measurements, or chest radiographs. Although relatively difficult to perform, PFTs provide excellent information about the status of an infant's lungs. Because of their sensitivity to minute physiologic changes, PFTs can detect alterations in an infant's status more reliably than other assessment techniques. Most of our observations on the effects of bronchodilators and diuretics on infants with BPD are based on PFT results.

Infants with BPD have significantly worse pulmonary function than either normal infants or infants who have recovered from respiratory distress syndrome.[2] Some of the pulmonary function abnormalities reported in infants with BPD include increased respiratory rate, increased minute ventilation, increased airway resistance (Raw), increased thoracic gas volume (TGV), decreased dynamic compliance (Cdyn), decreased maximal expiratory flow at functional residual capacity ($\dot{V}$maxFRC), abnormal gas exchange, elevated oxygen consumption, and increased work of breathing.[3-10] Table 1 lists the

**FIGURE 1 ■ An infant in the whole body pressure plethysmograph, used to measure thoracic gas volume (TGV), airways resistance (Raw), and tidal volume.**

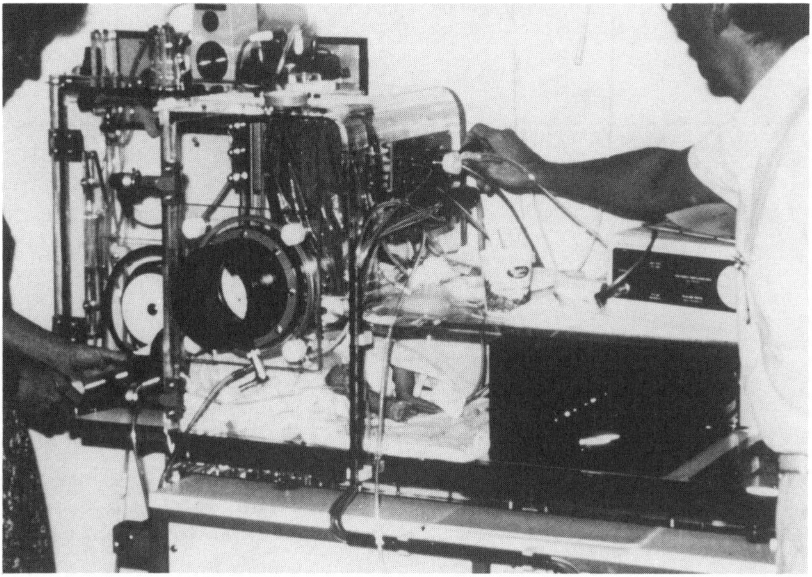

most common PFTs, what they measure, and the abnormalities they show in infants with BPD. We use the whole body pressure plethysmograph to measure respiratory rate, flow, tidal volume, TGV, and Raw (see Figure 1). An air-filled balloon is used to measure Cdyn (Figure 2), and rapid thoracoabdominal compression technique (or "Baby Hugger") measures $\dot{V}maxFRC$ (Figures 2 and 3).

## Diuretics

Diuretics were among the first agents tried in infants with BPD, and they remain the mainstay of pharmacologic treatment.[11]

Clinical, radiographic, and pathologic evidence show that a prominent feature of BPD is pulmonary edema. Pathologic studies in infants with BPD have demonstrated the presence of interstitial pulmonary edema, intra-alveolar edema, increased total lung water content, and dilated lymphatics.[12,13] Pulmonary congestion and edema may cause abnormalities of the small airways, characterized by increased flow resistance and premature airway closure. These in turn cause abnormalities of distribution of ventilation, resulting in the impaired gas exchange typical of BPD.[14]

**FIGURE 2 ■ An infant in the "Baby Hugger."** An air-filled balloon, passed into the esophagus, is used to measure dynamic compliance (Cdyn).

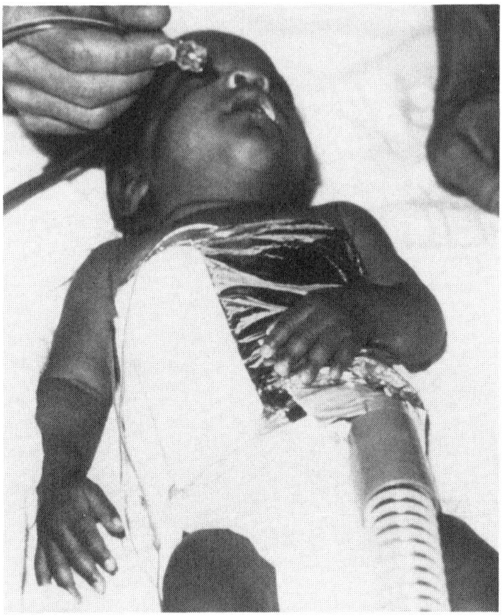

Because of the significance of edema in the pathophysiology of BPD, diuretics were one of the first pharmacologic modalities used for its treatment.[11,15] It is now clear that both oral and intravenous diuretics improve the pulmonary function and the clinical status of acutely ill infants with BPD.[2,15–17] The effect of diuretics is so dramatic that they are the most commonly used medications in infants with BPD, both in our nursery and in other nurseries throughout the country.[15–19]

Administration of intravenous furosemide (Lasix) to infants with ventilator dependent BPD produces a significant improvement in their minute ventilation, alveolar ventilation, and Cdyn, and it facilitates weaning from ventilatory support and supplemental oxygen.[15] Administration of intravenous furosemide also significantly decreases the degree of clinically evident respiratory distress in infants with BPD and improves their blood gases.[18]

We have shown that there is a rapid, short-term improvement in the pulmonary function tests of infants with BPD following the administration of furosemide. In a group of ten infants who were in the recovery phase of severe BPD, Raw decreased 36 percent, and Cdyn increased 54 percent from baseline within one hour after treatment with a single intravenous dose of furosemide.[2]

We have subsequently shown that a similar degree of improvement in PFT is seen in infants with BPD following a four-day course of oral chlorothiazide (Diuril) and spironolactone (Aldactone). Following treatment with these diuretics, Raw decreased 41 percent, and Cdyn increased 53 percent from baseline.[16]

The improvement of PFT in infants with BPD following treatment with diuretics is at least partly explained by diuresis and the subsequent removal of

**FIGURE 3 ■ Diagram of the rapid thoraco-abdominal compression technique, or "Baby Hugger" test;** measures maximal respiratory flow at functional residual capacity (VmaxFRC).

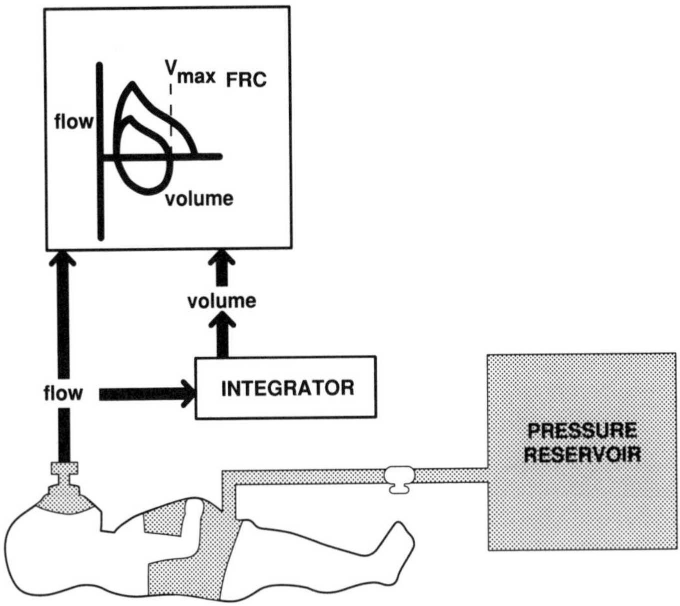


edema fluid from the pulmonary interstitium.[2,16,19] However, in animal models, these drugs also have nondiuretic actions on the lung. In animals, for example, furosemide increases lung lymph flow and lymph protein flow, decreases intrapulmonary shunt and pulmonary capillary leak, decreases pulmonary transvascular fluid filtration into the lungs, increases systemic and pulmonary venous capacity, and increases serum colloid osmotic pressure.[20–22] Both chlorothiazide and furosemide increase thoracic duct lymph flow.[20,23] The relative importance of the diuretic and nondiuretic actions of these agents in infants with BPD remains uncertain.

### Side Effects

Unfortunately, diuretics are not without side effects. Hyponatremia, hypokalemia, hypochloremia, and hypomagnesemia are all significant complications in patients who are treated with diuretics. Virtually all infants who are

**TABLE 2 ■ Dose Ranges for Diuretics Commonly Used in Infants with BPD at Children's Hospital, Oakland, California**

| MEDICATION | TRADE NAME | USUAL DOSAGE RANGE | ROUTE |
|---|---|---|---|
| Furosemide | Lasix | 1 mg/kg q 6–24 hours | IV/IM/PO |
| Spironolactone* | Aldactone | 1–2.5 mg/kg q 12 hours | PO |
| Chlorothiazide* | Diuril | 10–25 mg/kg q 12 hours | PO |

*Spironolactone and chlorothiazide usually administered simultaneously.

chronically treated with furosemide require supplemental electrolytes, usually as sodium chloride and/or potassium chloride.

Although the hyponatremia and hypokalemia are usually the more noticed effects of treatment with furosemide, hypochloremia is also of significant concern. One study in rabbits has shown that the chronic hypochloremic metabolic alkalosis that results from furosemide therapy can lead to a compensatory respiratory acidosis.[24] Although this is of theoretical concern, it has not been our impression that furosemide therapy is a significant cause of hypercarbia in our patients.

Another possible effect of hypochloremia is growth failure. This has not been shown to be a cause of growth failure in infants with BPD, but it is certainly a potential concern. One recent retrospective study of 23 infants who were hospitalized with severe BPD found that those infants who died were more likely to have significant hypochloremia than were those who survived.[25] Although this does not prove that hypochloremia caused or contributed to their death, it is of concern. It is our practice to maintain the chloride levels of all our infants above 90 mEq/liter.

Furosemide is also a potent calciuric agent. Because many infants with BPD also have suboptimal calcium stores, chronic treatment with furosemide can lead to severe osteopenia.[26] It is important to realize that, because of normal homeostatic control of calcium metabolism, serum calcium does not reflect whole-body calcium status; in fact, most infants with severe osteopenia will maintain a normal serum calcium level. In some infants treated with a prolonged course of intravenous furosemide, the resultant high urinary calcium levels can result in nephrolithiasis and nephrocalcinosis.[27] In contrast to furosemide, oral chlorothiazide appears to decrease renal calcium excretion and resolve established nephrolithiasis or nephrocalcinosis.[16,27]

The presence of calcium stones in the gall bladder (cholelithiasis) has also been described in infants receiving both parenteral nutrition and furosemide.[28] One report describes three infants who developed secondary hyperparathyroidism as a result of their prolonged exposure to furosemide.[29]

Two other concerns about furosemide, at least theoretically, are ototoxicity and displacement of conjugated bilirubin from albumin. Furosemide is possibly an ototoxic agent, at least in adults and animals.[30] However, the question of whether it causes ototoxicity has never been answered in infants. Furosemide is also capable of displacing unconjugated bilirubin from albumin, although this does not seem to be clinically significant.[31]

### Clinical Management

The doses of diuretics we use are shown in Table 2. For those infants who are developing BPD, we usually begin a trial of diuretics at three to four weeks of age. If the infant improves clinically, we continue the diuretic(s); if the infant shows no clinical improvement, we discontinue the diuretic(s). The infant who does not improve with the first trial usually receives a second trial approximately one to two weeks later.

To minimize the complications associated with furosemide, we treat infants with oral chlorothiazide and spironolactone and discontinue furosemide as soon as they are tolerating enteral nutrition. This combination seems to cause less electrolyte imbalance than does furosemide. Theoretically, it also reduces the risk of osteopenia.

## Bronchodilators

Until recently, bronchodilators have not been widely used in the early management of infants with BPD. This is perhaps because of histologic and physiologic evidence from studies of normal infants showing that they have relatively little smooth muscle in their small airways and that they do not respond to inhaled bronchodilators.[32–34] It is important to emphasize that these studies were conducted on infants who did not have BPD.

In contrast to the small amount of smooth muscle in the airways of healthy infants, infants with BPD have bronchiolar smooth muscle hypertrophy and evidence of airway obstruction.[5,35–37] Pulmonary function abnormalities reported in these infants include increased Raw and increased TGV secondary to air trapping.[4,6] Clinical studies also show that children with BPD have a significant degree of bronchial hyper-reactivity or bronchospasm.[5,38] Airway reactivity has been demonstrated in infants as young as 12 days postnatally and as premature as 26 weeks gestation.[39] This suggests that infants with BPD are good candidates for treatment with bronchodilators.

Older infants with BPD often have episodes of recurrent wheezing, suggesting that they may be more prone to bronchitis, bronchiolitis, or asth-

**TABLE 3 ■ Dose Ranges for Theophylline Commonly Used in Infants with BPD at Children's Hospital, Oakland, California**

| DOSE | ROUTE | IDEAL SERUM LEVEL |
|---|---|---|
| Loading: 5–7 mg/kg<br>Maintenance: 2–4 mg/kg q 6–8 hours<br>Total daily: 8 + postnatal age (months) mg/kg | IV/PO | 10–20 μg/ml |

Dose modified for BPD by Nickerson from Nassif et al.[90,91]

ma.[5,40] Of interest is the fact that these infants often have a family history that suggests an increased incidence of reactive airway disease.[38,41,42]

## Methylxanthines

The use of methylxanthines to treat BPD is somewhat more controversial than is the use of diuretics. Rooklin and coworkers reported a trend toward decreased Raw and increased Cdyn at 2 and 24 hours after a single intravenous dose of theophylline in patients with BPD.[43] Theophylline levels in these infants ranged from 5 to 12 μg/ml. Infants older than 1 month of age showed no improvement in pulmonary function following theophylline therapy.

In contrast to Rooklin's study, we have shown that oral theophylline significantly decreases Raw, increases VmaxFRC, and increases Cdyn in older infants with BPD.[17] The infants in our study had serum theophylline levels between 12 and 18 μg/ml. Table 3 shows the doses.

The effect of theophylline as a smooth muscle relaxant may be due to its ability to enhance intracellular levels of cyclic AMP by inhibiting phosphodiesterase. There appears to be a relationship between cyclic AMP levels and the degree of smooth muscle relaxation in rabbits.[44] Theophylline has been shown to accelerate pulmonary maturation by increasing cyclic AMP levels.[45] Theophylline is also a mild diuretic and may improve pulmonary mechanics by its diuretic action. This effect is due to enhanced glomerular filtration as a result of vasodilation.[46]

Theophylline is not without side effects. Sleep disturbances, tachycardia, agitation, and vomiting have all been associated with toxic levels, usually greater than 20 μg/ml.[47] Even with theophylline levels in the therapeutic range, behavioral changes have been detected in some infants.[48]

Until recently, there has been some concern that theophylline increases the metabolic rates of patients with BPD, thereby increasing their already high oxygen consumption. We have recently completed a study that showed no increase in oxygen consumption of infants with BPD treated with theophylline.[49]

**TABLE 4 ■ Dose Ranges for Inhaled Beta-Adrenergic Bronchodilators Commonly Used in Infants with BPD at Children's Hospital, Oakland, California**

| Medication | Trade Name | Concentration | Amount Administered |
|---|---|---|---|
| Isoetharine | Bronkosol | 1% solution | 5 breaths q 4–6 hrs |
| Terbutaline | Brethine | 0.1% solution | 5 breaths q 4–6 hrs |
| Metaproterenol | Alupent | 1% solution | 15 breaths q 4–6 hrs |
| Albuterol | Proventil | 0.5% solution | 15 breaths q 4–6 hrs |
| Isoproterenol | Isuprel | 0.1% solution | 5 breaths q 4–6 hrs |
| Atropine* | — | — | 0.08 mg/kg q 4–6 hrs |
| Cromolyn* | Intal | 20 mg/2 ml | 1 ml q 4–6 hrs |

*The dose ranges for atropine and cromolyn are not yet well established in neonates. The use of these agents, particularly cromolyn, should be considered experimental.

### Beta-Adrenergic Agents

Beta-adrenergic drugs include isoetharine (Bronkosol), terbutaline (Brethine), metaproterenol (Alupent), albuterol (also known as salbutamol, Proventil), and isoproterenol (Isuprel). All these have been used as aerosols to treat bronchoconstriction in asthmatic children and adults. Table 4 shows the inhaled bronchodilator doses that can be used in treatment of infants with BPD.

Several clinical trials have evaluated the efficacy of these bronchodilator aerosols in infants with BPD. Motoyama and coworkers demonstrated significant improvement in forced vital capacity (FVC) and maximal expiratory flow at 25 percent of FVC 15 minutes after isoetherine aerosol in 32 infants with ventilator-dependent BPD.[39] Similarly, Sosulski and associates showed that subcutaneous terbutaline significantly improved pulmonary function in ventilated patients with BPD.[50]

Cabal and coworkers recently demonstrated significant improvement in Cdyn, Raw, tidal volume, and transcutaneous carbon dioxide 15 minutes following metaproterenol administration in 8 infants with ventilator-dependent BPD at a mean postnatal age of one month.[51] Wilkie and Bryan demonstrated significantly improved respiratory system compliance (Crs) and respiratory system resistance (Rrs), one hour following salbutamol inhalation in 17 infants with ventilator-dependent BPD.[52] Smyth and associates reported significant improvement in expiratory flow rates following salbutamol inhalation in 5 school-age children with BPD.[5]

We reported rapid short-term improvement in Raw and specific airway conductance (SGaw) in ten infants with BPD following isoproterenol inhalation. We speculated that isoproterenol, a beta-2 sympathomimetic agonist, may have directly stimulated the bronchial smooth muscle, leading to bronchodilation.[53]

Metaproterenol inhalation is associated with an onset of action within 15–30 minutes, similar to that of isoproterenol. In contrast to isoproterenol, metaproterenol treatment has distinct advantages in infants because of its longer duration of action and lesser association with concomitant tachycardia.[54] Studies comparing the efficacy of metaproterenol and isoproterenol in adults with bronchospastic disease have suggested that metaproterenol is the superior drug for reversing bronchospasm. It also appears to have fewer side effects and a longer duration of action than does isoproterenol.[54,55]

### Anticholinergic Agents

There is evidence that there is resting vagal tone throughout the tracheobronchial tree, including terminal units, in normal individuals.[56,57] Animal studies have shown that stimulation of the vagal branches leading to the lung results in bronchial constriction.[58] This parasympathetic bronchial constriction can be prevented by atropine.[59] Investigators have shown that administration of anticholinergic agents increases both SGaw and $\mathring{V}$maxFRC in normal subjects. They conclude that inhibition of vagal tone by anticholinergic agents results in the dilation of large and small airways.[56]

Atropine aerosol, an anticholinergic bronchodilator, has been used to treat children and adults with asthma or chronic obstructive pulmonary disease.[60–63] One investigator reported significant improvement in forced expiratory flow, Raw, and SGaw following atropine or isoproterenol inhalation in children with asthma.[61] In another study, 6 of 15 infants less than one year of age with bronchiolitis showed significant improvement in the work of breathing following treatment with ipratropium bromide, an anticholinergic agent.[64] Yet another study demonstrated a significant decrease in Rrs and an increase in Crs one hour following inhalation of ipratropium bromide in five infants with ventilator-dependent BPD.[52]

Inhaled atropine has its predominant effect on the central airways, whereas that of metaproterenol is mainly on the small airways. One would therefore postulate that these two agents would be synergistic.

Several studies of adult subjects have reported that the combination of an anticholinergic agent with a beta-adrenergic agent causes greater bronchodilation than does either agent alone.[60,65–67] This synergy may be related to their different sites of action. In contrast to these studies, at least one recent study of adults suggests there is no synergistic effect of beta-adrenergic and anticholinergic bronchodilators.[68]

We have recently completed a study comparing the effects of inhaled metaproterenol (a beta agent), inhaled atropine (an anticholinergic agent), and combined metaproterenol and atropine in infants with BPD. We found the two agents to be of equal effect in improving Raw and $\mathring{V}$maxFRC. Both agents caused maximal improvement within one to two hours after treatment. The duration of both agents was three to six hours. Neither agent had any significant effect on Cdyn or TGV. We were unable to show any synergistic effect of the two agents.[69]

Caution should be used in applying our observations to the large, heterogeneous population with chronic air flow obstruction. Our infants were not tested repeatedly, so we cannot be certain that the bronchodilatory effects we observed are consistent over time. Our results do not encourage the use of combination therapy, but they do not preclude the value of combinations of agents in certain subgroups of patients under special circumstances.

## Clinical Management

We have compared the effects of oral theophylline, oral diuretics, and combined oral theophylline and diuretics on the pulmonary function of infants with BPD.[17] This study showed that oral diuretics and theophylline have synergistic effects. Combined therapy with theophylline plus diuretics improved Raw, SGaw, Cdyn, and $\mathring{V}maxFRC$ significantly more than theophylline alone. Theophylline plus diuretics improved Cdyn significantly more than diuretics alone. However, of the two individual agents, the diuretics alone improved pulmonary function more than the theophylline alone. Based on these findings, we feel that it is appropriate to use diuretics plus theophylline in infants with severe BPD.

Ideally, inhaled beta agents should be ordered as 4 hourly treatments—not as 8–12 hourly or PRN treatments. It is clear that most of the effect of the beta agents is gone by 4 hours (possibly slightly longer with albuterol, although this has not been studied in newborns). It is also clear from experience with asthmatic patients that the beta agents are most effective when used on a regular schedule, rather than PRN. When an infant no longer requires treatments every 4 hours, we try to discontinue the treatments.

Ideally, treatments should be given to ventilated infants by "bagging" rather than "in line" with the ventilator. This is because much of the medication administered by the "in line" method is lost in the continuous flow rather than being delivered to the infant.

Extubated infants may receive their treatments as "blow-by" or continuous positive airway pressure, rather than as bagged breaths. No evidence suggests that the delivery of aerosols by positive pressure is more effective than by spontaneous ventilation.

The ideal administration technique of inhaled agents is probably with a metered dose inhaler. Although this is not well studied in infants, there is considerable evidence in both adults and children that these inhalers are a safe and effective tool for dispensing aerosol agents.

## Other Agents

In addition to diuretics and bronchodilators, a number of other pharmacologic agents have been used to decrease the incidence or lessen the severity of BPD. These agents should probably still be considered unproven in their efficacy.

### Cromolyn

This is a drug proven to be extremely useful for managing asthma in both adults and children.[70] Because it seems to block bronchoconstriction, it should theoretically be useful for managing some infants with BPD. We have used it only rarely. Our impression is that its efficacy is at best equivocal. The dose range is shown in Table 4.

### Steroids

The glucocorticoid group of steroids have multiple, diverse actions, many of which may be beneficial in the treatment of pulmonary disease.[71] They are used extensively to treat a broad range of disorders, including asthma and adult chronic obstructive pulmonary disease. As might be expected, steroids have also been used to treat infants with BPD.

Possible mechanisms of action include increased surfactant synthesis, stabilization of cell and lysosomal membranes, inhibition of prostaglandin and leukotriene synthesis, enhancement of prostaglandin $E_2$ breakdown, increased prostaglandin levels, decreased pulmonary and bronchial edema, decreased bronchospasm, decreased polymorphonuclear leukocyte recruitment to lungs, breakdown of polymorphonuclear leukocyte aggregates in the pulmonary microcirculation, and enhancement of beta-adrenergic activity.[71]

In a small controlled trial of dexamethasone in a group of infants who continued to need ventilation at four weeks of age despite maximal therapy with diuretics and bronchodilators, the steroid-treated group showed a significantly decreased need for ventilatory support.[72] However, two-thirds of the infants treated with dexamethasone developed sepsis. Other side effects of steroid therapy include systemic hypertension, glucose instability, growth failure, and pneumothorax (due to the sudden improvement in compliance and failure to wean ventilation rapidly).

A trial of dexamethasone in infants who were younger (two to four weeks of age) showed that dexamethasone improved the status of infants with mild BPD but not of those with established cystic changes.[73] This study failed to confirm a high incidence of sepsis.

The efficacy of steroids in improving Cdyn in infants with early BPD was confirmed in a study by Avery and coworkers.[74] As they pointed out, however, little is known about the long-term effects of treating growing premature infants with steroids. Steroids should probably not yet be considered routine therapy for infants with BPD.

A multicenter trial of steroids for the treatment of BPD is currently in progress in Great Britain. Hopefully, this will provide us with more information about which infants are most likely to benefit from steroids.

### Antioxidants

Oxygen, in concentrations above that found in room air, can cause significant pulmonary toxicity, at least in the mature lung.[75] There is probably also a component of oxygen toxicity in BPD.[76] It therefore makes sense to attempt to prevent or reduce the severity of BPD with antioxidants.

The mammalian body is equipped with a complex system for decreasing oxidant injury, one aspect of which is the enzyme superoxide dismutase (SOD). Levels of this enzyme seem to be lower in preterm infants with hyaline membrane disease than in those without it. Furthermore, infants who recover from hyaline membrane disease without developing BPD have higher SOD levels than infants who develop BPD.[77] This does not show a causal relationship, but it led to several clinical trials of the effect of SOD on the incidence of BPD. Parenteral SOD appears to be safe.[78] In one study of 45 infants at risk for BPD, the subcutaneous administration of SOD decreased the clinical and radiographic incidence of BPD, although it did not alter the duration of either mechanical ventilation or supplemental oxygen.[79] These results must be interpreted with caution, and SOD therapy should still be considered experimental.[80]

Superoxide dismutase is not the only antioxidant that has been used in an attempt to decrease the incidence of BPD. Vitamin E is also known to be a potent blocker of oxidant injury.[81] Not surprisingly, its effects on the course of BPD have been investigated. Also not surprising are the divergent results of these studies. In a study of 40 premature infants with hyaline membrane disease, those treated with intramuscular vitamin E injections had a barely significantly lower incidence of BPD.[82] However, a similar study was unable to demonstrate any significant difference between placebo and vitamin E treated infants in the incidence of BPD.[83] Currently, we do not feel that there is a role for the routine treatment of infants with vitamin E, other than to maintain physiologic levels.

### Vitamin A

Recently attention has focused on vitamin A deficiency in premature infants and its possible causal role in the development of BPD. In a study of almost 100 preterm infants, two-thirds had low vitamin A levels, suggesting deficiency.[84] In this and in another similar study, those infants who developed BPD had significantly lower vitamin A levels than those who did not.[85]

The only controlled trial of vitamin A supplementation for preventing BPD showed that intramuscular vitamin A, when given to infants every other day for the first month of life, led to a significant decrease in the incidence of BPD.[86] One possible explanation for this is that, at least in adult mice, vitamin A deficiency worsens oxygen toxicity.[87]

Again, these results should be viewed as preliminary, and the use of pharmacologic doses of vitamin A should be regarded as experimental.

## Clinical Management of Pharmacologic Intervention

We consider diuretics to be our first line of therapy for infants with BPD. We usually begin treatment when an infant is one month old and has clinical and radiographic evidence of significant BPD, although in some cases, we begin earlier. We continue diuretics until the infant no longer requires either ventilatory support or supplemental oxygen. We suspect that some infants with BPD may continue to benefit from diuretics even after they have been weaned to room air, although this has never been proven. We are currently conducting a controlled study to answer this question.

Because many of the smallest infants with BPD are not taking enteral nutrition, our first diuretic is often intravenous furosemide. However, furosemide has significant side effects, particularly hypercalciuria, hyponatremia, hypokalemia, and hypochloremia. Oral therapy with furosemide is less effective because it is poorly absorbed in infants of this age.[88,89] For these reasons, we switch to oral spironolactone and chlorothiazide when infants are tolerating enteral feeding. We use the combination of spironolactone and chlorothiazide because of their synergy and because of the potassium-sparing effect of spironolactone.

Our second line of therapy is bronchodilators. Because of theophylline toxicity, we tend to treat infants initially with inhaled beta-adrenergic agents. Only if they do not respond adequately do we either change to theophylline or add it to the beta-agonists. We virtually never treat infants with bronchodilators unless they are also receiving diuretics. We also tend to discontinue the bronchodilators before we discontinue the diuretics. The use of anticholinergic bronchodilators is less routine, largely because most infants respond as well or better to the beta-agonists.

## Unanswered Questions

Despite all we know about the effects of drugs on the course of infants with BPD, there are many more questions than answers about the optimal management of these infants. Some of the questions we hope to see answered in the next several years include:

1. How early in the course of BPD are diuretics and bronchodilators effective? Does early treatment with diuretics and/or bronchodilators alter the long-term course of BPD? Most research to date has focused on infants more than one month of age, although many people administer these medications empirically to younger infants.
2. What is the relative efficacy of inhaled bronchodilators and diuretics? Are they synergistic in the same way that theophylline and diuretics are?
3. Are inhaled bronchodilators more or less effective than theophylline? Are they synergistic with theophylline?
4. How long should diuretics and/or bronchodilators be continued—until the infant is off the ventilator, off oxygen, or ready for school?
5. Do steroids really work? If so, for which infants? What is the optimal dose and timing?
6. Is there a clinical role for antioxidants, vitamin A supplementation, or cromolyn?
7. Perhaps most important, what are the long-term side effects of administering all these agents to infants?

## References


1. Kao LC, et al.: Reproducibility of pulmonary function in infants with bronchopulmonary dysplasia, American Review of Respiratory Diseases 133, 1986, p. A208.
2. Kao LC, et al.: Furosemide acutely decreases airway resistance in chronic bronchopulmonary dysplasia, Journal of Pediatrics 103, 1983, pp. 624–629.
3. Durand M, and Rigatto H: Tidal volume and respiratory frequency in infants with bronchopulmonary dysplasia (BPD), Early Human Development 5, 1981, pp. 55–62.
4. Morray JP, et al.: Improvement in lung mechanics as a function of age in the infant with severe bronchopulmonary dysplasia, Pediatric Research 16, 1982, pp. 290–294.
5. Smyth JA, et al.: Pulmonary function and bronchial hyperreactivity in long-term survivors of bronchopulmonary dysplasia, Pediatrics 68, 1981, pp. 336–340.
6. Watts JL, Ariagno RL, and Brady JP: Chronic pulmonary disease in neonates after artificial ventilation: Distribution of ventilation and pulmonary interstitial emphysema, Pediatrics 60, 1977, pp. 273–281.
7. Lindroth M, et al.: Pulmonary mechanics, chest x-ray and lung disease after mechanical ventilation in low birth weight infants, Acta Paediatrica Scandinavica 69, 1980, pp. 761–770.

8. Godfrey S, et al.: Flow-volume curves in infants with lung disease, Pediatrics 72, 1983, pp. 517–522.
9. Weinstein MR, and Oh W: Oxygen consumption in infants with bronchopulmonary dysplasia, Journal of Pediatrics 99, 1981, pp. 958–961.
10. Wolfson MR, et al.: Mechanics and energetics of breathing helium in infants with bronchopulmonary dysplasia, Journal of Pediatrics 104, 1984, pp. 752–757.
11. Sniderman S, et al.: Treatment of neonatal chronic lung disease with furosemide, Pediatric Research 15, 1981, p. A682.
12. O'Brodovich HM, and Mellins RB: Bronchopulmonary dysplasia, unresolved neonatal acute lung injury, American Review of Respiratory Diseases 132, 1985, pp. 694–700.
13. Northway WH, Rosan RC, and Porter DY: Pulmonary disease following respiratory therapy of hyaline-membrane disease: Bronchopulmonary dysplasia, New England Journal of Medicine 276, 1967, pp. 357–368.
14. Milic-Emili J, and Ruff F: Effects of pulmonary congestion and edema on the small airways, Bulletin of European Physiopathology of Respiration 7, 1971, pp. 1181–1196.
15. McCann EM, et al.: Controlled trial of furosemide therapy in infants with chronic lung disease, Journal of Pediatrics 106, 1985, pp. 957–962.
16. Kao LC, et al.: Effect of oral diuretics on pulmonary mechanics in infants with chronic bronchopulmonary dysplasia: Results of a double-blind crossover sequential trial, Pediatrics 74, 1984, pp. 37–44.
17. Kao LC, et al.: Oral theophylline and diuretics improve pulmonary mechanics in infants with bronchopulmonary dysplasia, Journal of Pediatrics 111, 1987, pp. 439–444.
18. Engelhardt B, Elliott S, and Hazinski TA: Short- and long-term effects of furosemide on lung function in infants with bronchopulmonary dysplasia, Journal of Pediatrics 109, 1986, pp. 1034–1039.
19. O'Donovan BH, and Bell EF: Effects of furosemide on body water compartments in infants with bronchopulmonary dysplasia, Pediatric Research 26, 1989, pp. 121–124.
20. Szwed JJ, Kleit SA, and Hamburger RJ: Effect of furosemide and chlorothiazide on the thoracic duct lymph flow in the dog, Journal of Laboratory Clinical Medicine 79, 1972, pp. 693–700.
21. Ali J, Chernicki W, and Wood LDH: Effect of furosemide in canine low-pressure pulmonary edema, Journal of Clinical Investigation 64, 1979, pp. 1494–1504.
22. Bland RD, McMillan DD, and Bressack MA: Decreased pulmonary transvascular fluid filtration in awake newborn lambs after intravenous furosemide, Journal of Clinical Investigation 62, 1978, pp. 601–609.
23. McCaffrey C, and Levy M: Effect of furosemide on the thoracic duct lymph flow in the dog, American Journal of Physiology 238, 1980, pp. 363–371.
24. Hazinski TA: Furosemide decreases ventilation in young rabbits, Journal of Pediatrics 106, 1985, pp. 81–85.
25. Perlman JM, et al.: Is chloride depletion an important contributing cause of death in infants with bronchopulmonary dysplasia? Pediatrics 77, 1986, pp. 212–216.
26. Ryan S, et al.: Bone mineral content in bronchopulmonary dysplasia, Archives of Disease in Childhood 62, 1987, pp. 889–894.

27. Hufnagle KG, et al.: Renal calcifications: A complication of long-term furosemide therapy in preterm infants, Pediatrics 70, 1982, pp. 360–363.
28. Whitington PG, and Black DD: Cholelithiasis in premature infants treated with parenteral nutrition and furosemide, Journal of Pediatrics 97, 1980, pp. 647–649.
29. Venkataraman PS, et al.: Secondary hyperparathyroidism and bone disease in infants receiving long-term furosemide therapy, American Journal of Diseases of Children 137, 1983, pp. 1157–1161.
30. Rybak LP: Furosemide ototoxicity: Clinical and experimental aspects, Laryngoscope 95 (supplement 38), 1985, pp. 1–14.
31. Broderson R: Bilirubin transport in the newborn infant, reviewed with relation to kernicterus, Journal of Pediatrics 96, 1980, pp. 349–356.
32. Matsuko K, and Thurlbeck WM: A morphometric study of bronchial and bronchiolar walls in children, American Review of Respiratory Disease 105, 1972, pp. 908–913.
33. Rutter N, Milner AD, and Hiller EF: Effect of bronchodilators on respiratory resistance in infants and young children with bronchiolitis and wheezy bronchitis, Archives of Disease in Childhood 50, 1975, pp. 719–722.
34. Lenny W, and Milner AD: At what age do bronchodilator drugs work? Archives of Disease in Childhood 53, 1978, pp. 532–535.
35. Bonikos DS, et al.: Bronchopulmonary dysplasia: The pulmonary pathologic sequel of necrotizing bronchiolitis and pulmonary fibrosis, Human Pathology 7, 1976, pp. 643–666.
36. Borkenstein J, Borkenstein M, and Rosegger H: Pulmonary function studies in long-term survivors with artificial ventilation in the neonatal period, Acta Paediatrica Scandinavica 69, 1980, pp. 159–163.
37. Rosan RC: Hyaline membrane disease and a related spectrum of neonatal pneumopathies, Perspectives in Pediatric Pathology 2, 1975, pp. 15–60.
38. Nickerson BG, and Taussig LM: Family history of asthma in infants with bronchopulmonary dysplasia, Pediatrics 65, 1980, pp. 1140–1144.
39. Motoyama EK, et al.: Early onset of airway reactivity in premature infants with bronchopulmonary dysplasia, American Review of Respiratory Disease 136, 1987, pp. 50–57.
40. Johnson JO, et al.: Prognosis of children surviving with the aid of mechanical ventilation in the newborn period, Journal of Pediatrics 84, 1974, pp. 272–276.
41. Bertrand JM, et al.: The long-term pulmonary sequelae of prematurity: The role of familial airway hyperactivity and the respiratory distress syndrome, New England Journal of Medicine 312, 1985, pp. 742–745.
42. Fineberg M, et al.: Bronchial hyperreactivity in parents of infants with bronchopulmonary dysplasia, American Review of Respiratory Disease 131, 1985, p. A265.
43. Rooklin AR, et al.: Theophylline therapy in bronchopulmonary dysplasia, Journal of Pediatrics 95, 1979, pp. 882–885.
44. Anderson RGG: Cyclic AMP and calcium ions in mechanical and metabolic responses of smooth muscles: Influence of some hormones and drugs, Acta Paediatrica Scandinavica 382 (supplement), 1972, pp. 1–59.

45. Barrett CT, et al.: Effects of cortisol and aminophylline upon survival, pulmonary mechanics, and secreted phosphatidyl choline of prematurely delivered rabbits, Pediatric Research 12, 1978, pp. 38–42.
46. Kover G, Tost H, and Stimacz E: Effect of cyclic 3′ 5′ adenosine monophosphate and theophylline on renal function, Acta Physiologica Academiae Scientiarum Hungaricae 42, 1972, pp. 111–117.
47. Howell J, Clozel M, and Aranda JV: Adverse effects of caffeine and theophylline in the newborn infant, Seminars in Perinatology 5, 1981, pp. 359–368.
48. Loisel DB, Smith MM, and MacDonald MG: Plasma theophylline levels as related to toxicity in infants with severe chronic lung disease, Neonatal Network 6(2), 1987, pp. 15–19.
49. Kao LC, Durand DJ, and Nickerson BG: Improving pulmonary function does not decrease oxygen consumption in infants with bronchopulmonary dysplasia, Journal of Pediatrics 112, 1988, pp. 616–621.
50. Sosulski R, et al.: Physiologic effects of terbutaline on pulmonary function of infants with bronchopulmonary dysplasia, Pediatric Pulmonology 2, 1986, pp. 269–273.
51. Cabal L, et al.: Effects of metaproterenol on pulmonary mechanics, oxygenation, and ventilation in infants with chronic lung disease, Journal of Pediatrics 110, 1987, pp. 116–119.
52. Wilkie RA, and Bryan MH: Effect of bronchodilators on airway resistance in ventilator-dependent neonates with chronic lung disease, Journal of Pediatrics 111, 1987, pp. 278–282.
53. Kao LC, et al.: Effect of isoproterenol inhalation on airway resistance in chronic bronchopulmonary dysplasia, Pediatrics 73, 1984, pp. 509–514.
54. Fairshter RD, and Wilson AF: Response to inhaled metaproterenol and isoproterenol in asthmatic and normal subjects, Chest 73, 1980, pp. 44–50.
55. Sobol BJ, and Reed A: The rapidity of onset of bronchodilation: A comparison of alupent and isoproterenol, Annals of Allergy 32, 1974, pp. 137–141.
56. Douglas NJ, Sudlow MF, and Flenley DC: Effect of an inhaled atropine-like agent on normal airway function, Journal of Applied Physiology 46, 1979, pp. 256–262.
57. DeTroyer A, Yernault JC, and Rodensten D: Effects of vagal blockade on lung mechanics in normal man, Journal of Applied Physiology 46, 1979, pp. 217–226.
58. Colebach HJH, and Halmagyi DFJ: Effect of vagotomy and vagal stimulation on lung mechanics and circulation, Journal of Applied Physiology 18, 1963, pp. 881–887.
59. Vincent NJ, et al.: Factors influencing pulmonary resistance, Journal of Applied Physiology 29, 1970, pp. 236–243.
60. Bruderman I, Cohen-Aronovski R, and Smorzik J: A comparative study of various combinations of ipratropium bromide and metaproterenol in allergic asthmatic patients, Chest 83, 1983, pp. 208–210.
61. Cropp GJA: The role of parasympathetic nervous system in the maintenance of chronic airway obstruction in asthmatic children, American Review of Respiratory Disease 112, 1975, pp. 599–605.
62. Klock LE, et al.: A comparative study of atropine sulfate and isoproterenol hydrochloride in chronic bronchitis, American Review of Respiratory Disease 112, 1975, pp. 371–376.

63. Marini JJ, and Lakshminarayan S: The effect of atropine inhalation in "irreversible" chronic bronchitis, Chest 77, 1980, pp. 591–596.
64. Stokes GM, et al.: Nebulized therapy in acute severe bronchiolitis in infancy, Archives of Diseases in Childhood 58, 1983, pp. 279–283.
65. Petrie GR, and Palmer KNV: Comparison of aerosol ipratropium bromide and salbutamol in chronic bronchitis and asthma, British Medical Journal 1, 1975, pp. 430–432.
66. Gross NJ, and Skorodin MS: Anticholinergic, antimuscarinic bronchodilators, American Review of Respiratory Disease 129, 1984, pp. 856–870.
67. Lightbody IM, et al.: Ipratropium bromide, salbutamol and prednisolone in bronchial asthma and chronic bronchitis, British Journal of Diseases of the Chest 72, 1978, pp. 517–522.
68. Easton PA, et al.: A comparison of the bronchodilating effects of a beta-adrenergic agent (albuterol) and an anticholinergic agent (ipratropium bromide), given by aerosol alone or in sequence, New England Journal of Medicine 315, 1986, pp. 735–739.
69. Kao LC, et al.: Metaproterenol and atropine aerosols improve pulmonary mechanics in infants with bronchopulmonary dysplasia (BPD), Pediatric Pulmonology 6, 1989, pp. 74–80.
70. Berstein IL: Cromolyn sodium, Chest 87 (supplement), 1985, pp. 68S–72S.
71. Morris HG: Mechanisms of glucocorticoid action in pulmonary disease, Chest 88, 1985, pp. 133S–141S.
72. Mammel MC, et al.: Controlled trial of dexamethasone therapy in infants with bronchopulmonary dysplasia, Lancet 2, 1983, pp. 1356–1358.
73. Barrington K, and Finer NN: Evaluation of the efficacy of dexamethasone in prevention of severe bronchopulmonary dysplasia, Journal of Perinatology 5, 1985, pp. 26–32.
74. Avery GB, et al.: Controlled trial of dexamethasone in respirator-dependent infants with bronchopulmonary dysplasia, Pediatrics 75, 1985, pp. 106–111.
75. Deneke S, and Fanburg B: Normobaric oxygen toxicity of the lung, New England Journal of Medicine 303, 1980, pp. 76–86.
76. Phillip AGS: Oxygen plus pressure plus time: The etiology of bronchopulmonary dysplasia, Pediatrics 55, 1975, pp. 44–50.
77. Bonta BW, Gawron ER, and Warshaw JB: Neonatal red cell superoxide dismutase enzyme levels: Possible role as a cellular defense mechanism against pulmonary oxygen toxicity, Pediatric Research 11, 1977, pp. 754–757.
78. Rosenfeld W, et al.: Safety and plasma concentrations of bovine superoxide dismutase administered to human premature infants, Developmental Pharmacological Therapy 5, 1982, pp. 151–161.
79. Rosenfield W, et al.: Prevention of bronchopulmonary dysplasia by administration of bovine superoxide dismutase in preterm infants with respiratory distress syndrome, Journal of Pediatrics 105, 1984, pp. 781–785.
80. Gerdes JS: Superoxide dismutase in prevention of bronchopulmonary dysplasia (letter), Journal of Pediatrics 106, 1985, p. 1057.
81. Gleason CG, and Carlo WA: Vitamin E and the newborn infant: The shady lady reborn, Journal of Perinatology 5, 1985, pp. 21–27.

82. Ehrenkranz RA, et al.: Amelioration of bronchopulmonary dysplasia after vitamin E administration: A preliminary report, New England Journal of Medicine 299, 1978, pp. 564–569.
83. Saldanha RL, Cepeda EE, and Poland RL: The effect of vitamin E prophylaxis on the incidence and severity of bronchopulmonary dysplasia, Journal of Pediatrics 101, 1982, pp. 89–93.
84. Hustead VA, et al.: Relationship of vitamin A (retinol) status to lung disease in the preterm infant, Journal of Pediatrics 105, 1984, pp. 610–615.
85. Shenai JP, Chytil F, and Stahlman MT: Vitamin A status of neonates with bronchopulmonary dysplasia, Pediatric Research 19, 1985, pp. 185–189.
86. Shenai JP, et al.: Clinical trial of vitamin A supplementation in infants susceptible to bronchopulmonary dysplasia, Journal of Pediatrics 111, 1987, pp. 269–277.
87. Cohen-Addad N, et al.: Vitamin A deficiency and pulmonary oxygen toxicity: Morphometric studies in the murine lung, Pediatric Research 23, 1988, pp. 76–80.
88. Peterson RG, et al.: Pharmacology of furosemide in the premature newborn infant, Journal of Pediatrics 97, 1980, pp. 139–143.
89. Mirochnick MH, et al.: Furosemide pharmacokinetics in very low birth weight infants, Journal of Pediatrics 112, 1988, pp. 653–657.
90. Nickerson BG: Bronchopulmonary dysplasia: Chronic pulmonary disease following neonatal respiratory failure, Chest 87, 1985, pp. 528–535.
91. Nassif EG, et al.: Theophylline disposition in infancy, Journal of Pediatrics 98, 1981, pp. 158–161.

## CHAPTER 5

# Nutrition and Bronchopulmonary Dysplasia

*Carolyn Lund, RN, MS*
*Children's Hospital,*
*Oakland, California*
*Sharon Boatright Collier, RD*
*Children's Hospital,*
*Boston, Massachusetts*

Optimal nutrition is essential to infants with bronchopulmonary dysplasia (BPD) to permit tissue repair and overall organ growth as they begin to "outgrow" their lung disease. Nutrition is also a key factor in promoting normal development in infancy, and must be provided for these infants if they are to reach their full potential. However, providing nutrition to BPD infants is difficult because of the constraints surrounding their disease state and relative organ immaturity. In this chapter, nutritional goals, problems and controversies for BPD infants throughout the course of their initial hospitalization will be explored. Strategies for improving nutritional outcome are presented relative to the stage of illness.

In discussing nutritional care for infants with BPD, this article borrows a classification used by William Oh, MD, in a recent Ross Roundtable.[1] The specific stages of nutritional concerns are presented in the following order: acute stage nutritional management (the intubated infant on total parenteral nutrition), intermediate stage nutritional management (the intubated infant progressing toward an enteral diet), and chronic stage nutritional management (establishing oral feeds in the stable infant on nasal cannula, hood oxygen, or with a tracheostomy).

## Acute Stage

During the early days of hospitalization, the premature infant with respiratory distress syndrome (RDS) and also some term infants with meconium aspiration, pneumonias, and other lung diseases are at high risk of developing some degree of BPD. The following guidelines are applicable to prematures in general but may be even more critical for the very ill infant who later develops moderate to severe chronic lung disease.

### Fluid Management

Meticulous fluid management is necessary for all infants with RDS during the early stages of hospitalization. The combination of overhydration and mechanical ventilation is likely to leave residual lung damage in infants with RDS.[2] The findings of one study suggest that, despite strict surveillance to prevent overhydration, certain infants were less able to excrete body water. This absence of the "diuretic phase" of RDS during the first 72 hours of life placed them at higher risk for the development of BPD.[3] Similar to the increased incidence of BPD in infants with overhydration, infants with a patent ductus arteriosus (PDA) resulting in pulmonary edema show an increased incidence of BPD. The presence of excess pulmonary fluid has been identified as the second stage in the pathogenesis of BPD.[4]

Providing adequate hydration without fluid overload remains a constant challenge in the care of the very low-birthweight infant at high risk for BPD. Initial fluid rates, generally 55–70 cc/kg/day, are gradually increased to 80–150 cc/kg/day during the first week as the infant's lung condition improves and excess total body water is excreted. It is not unusual to see a weight loss of 10–15 percent of birthweight during this time. However, losses for some infants can be even more dramatic, placing them in jeopardy from dehydration.

Extreme insensible water losses, primarily through very immature skin, can rapidly dehydrate the tiny premature infant. This tendency toward dehydration is magnified by the use of a radiant warming table for thermoregulation or the use of phototherapy. Some infants can require fluid levels of 200–400 cc/kg/day in order to maintain a normal serum sodium level, normal urine output, and adequate blood pressure. Providing fluids at this level creates a dilemma because of the danger of overhydration as shifts in water balance occur.

Measures to reduce the amount of insensible water losses and control fluid balance, such as the use of double-walled incubators, plastic wrap, and humidity, can be introduced during the early phase of hospitalization.[5-7] Measures of hydration status—body weight, serum sodium, urine output, and specific gravity—require close monitoring. Overhydration is another concern

**TABLE 1 ■ Estimated Energy Requirements (kcal/kg/day) for Infants in Each Stage of BPD**

| COMPONENT | ACUTE PHASE | INTERMEDIATE PHASE | CONVALESCENT PHASE |
|---|---|---|---|
| Basal metabolic rate (BMR) | 45 | 60 | 60 |
| Stool losses | 0–10 | 10 | 10 |
| Thermal stress | 0–10 | 0–10 | 10 |
| Activity | 5 | 5 | 10 |
| Specific dynamic action (SDA) | 0 | 0–5 | 10 |
| Growth | 0 | 20–30 | 20–30 |
| Total (kcal/kg/day) | 50–70 | 95–120 | 120–130 |

From: 90th Ross Conference on Pediatric Research, p. 98. Reprinted by permission of Ross Laboratories, Columbus, Ohio 43216.

and requires looking at fluid intake data as well. Optimal care requires that hydration be achieved at fluid administration of less than 150 cc/kg/day. This is extremely difficult in the very low-birthweight infant with significant insensible water losses. Fortunately, this period of extreme insensible water loss is limited to the first 10–14 days of life; after this time, the skin matures and can more efficiently prevent water loss.

## Nutritional Requirements

The nutritional and caloric goals during the early phase of illness in infants likely to develop BPD are primarily to provide enough calories to meet the basal metabolic rate (BMR) and avoid tissue breakdown. Growth is not expected during this time; in fact, a weight loss of up to 10 percent is more typically seen.

The basal metabolic rate refers to the amount of energy necessary to maintain basic body functions such as respiratory, cardiac, and renal activity. Table 1 shows the components of energy expenditure that contribute to an estimated requirement of 50–70 kcal/kg/day during this acute stage. During the intermediate and chronic stages, the caloric requirement increases as growth, tissue repair, and the development of muscle mass occurs.

**Protein.** Protein requirements during this acute stage reflect the need to maintain basic body functions and avoid catabolism, or a state of negative nitrogen balance. There are limited body stores of protein. In the absence of adequate protein calorie intake, the premature utilizes muscle protein for gluconeogenesis. An intake of 60 non-nitrogen kcal/kg/day and

2.5 gm/kg/day of amino acids has been shown to put premature infants into positive nitrogen balance. In the small preterm or very ill infant, higher amounts of protein, at least 2.5–3 gm/kg/day, are required to promote growth of new tissue, and some evidence suggests that 3–3.5 gm/kg/day might better meet the needs for growth and tissue repair in these infants.[8]

If protein is provided without adequate amounts of carbohydrate and fat calories, however, a negative or inappropriate ratio of protein calories to nonprotein calories develops. The ratio of protein to nonprotein calories should be at least 1:24–40. (This means that for every gram of protein provided there should be 24–40 calories provided as fat or carbohydrate; this ratio is sometimes expressed as nonprotein calories/gm nitrogen and should be 150–200:1.)[9] If the amount of protein delivered exceeds this ratio, protein will be used (very inefficiently) as an energy source rather than for tissue repair and growth, and elevated serum ammonia levels may result.

**Fat.** Fat calories are utilized during the acute stage of illness to prevent essential fatty acid deficiency and to provide a source of calories that minimizes fluid intake. Intravenous fat emulsion (IVF) provides an excellent source of nonprotein calories with minimal fluid intake: 10 percent IVF provides 1.1 kcal/ml; 20 percent IVF contains 2 kcal/ml.

IVF contains linoleic acid, an essential fatty acid important in brain myelination, prostaglandin metabolism, and platelet function. Without provision of IVF, the premature infant rapidly develops biochemical evidence of essential fatty acid deficiency. After several weeks, clinical symptoms begin, including a scaly dermatitis and platelet dysfunction. A dose of 0.5–1 gm/kg/day of IVF is sufficient to prevent essential fatty acid deficiency.[10]

Several complicating factors may enter into the decision to use intravenous fats in the early stages of care. Significant hyperbilirubinemia is a contraindication to providing more than a minimal dose of intravenous fats since fatty acids are released when IVF is hydrolyzed and may displace bilirubin from albumin and increase the risk of kernicterus.[11,12]

Concerns have also been raised about the effect of IVF on diffusion of oxygen in the blood and on blood pH. A recent study indicated that in prematures weighing less than 1,500 gm, the rate of IVF infusion was likely the most critical factor. When IVF was delivered as a constant infusion over a 24-hour period (at a rate not exceeding 0.17 gm/kg/hour), a dose as high as 4 gm/kg/day could safely be tolerated in terms of pulmonary and blood pH stability.[13] Most neonatal units limit the dose of IVF to 3 gm/kg/day at a slower infusion rate. In general, a continuous lipid infusion is preferred over an intermittent regimen.[14]

Most investigators agree that the number of calories supplied to an individual infant as fat should not exceed 60 percent of the total intake, as more than this may result in ketosis. IVF administration can cause hyperlipidemia, a fat overload syndrome characterized by massive hypertriglyceridemia and disseminated intravascular coagulation. Methods for monitoring the safe and efficient utilization of intravenous fat are controversial, however. The method of visually inspecting serum for turbidity (obtaining a capillary tube of blood, spinning a hematocrit, and looking at the serum portion for evidence of cloudiness) has been shown to be inaccurate.[15] Another method, nephelometry, has not been found to be useful in monitoring IVF overdosage.[16] Triglyceride and cholesterol levels provide a better indication of IVF tolerance. Triglyceride levels less than 150–200 mg/dl and cholesterol levels less than 250 mg/dl are generally accepted as safe levels for these infants.[9]

**Carbohydrates.** The most widely utilized source of calories for infants during the acute stage of illness, as RDS progresses to BPD, is carbohydrate supplied as intravenous glucose. Usually initiated within hours of birth to prevent hypoglycemia, intravenous glucose provides most or all of the calories for these infants during the first days of life.

Because a 10 percent glucose solution contains 34 calories per 100 ml of fluid, providing the majority of calories in this way also means providing a significant amount of fluid.[9] To meet the basal metabolic requirement of 50 kcal/kg/day, a 1,000 gm infant would need at least 148 cc/kg/day of 10 percent dextrose in water. This level of fluid intake may be excessive for many infants with RDS and may increase the risk of developing PDA or BPD. Also, many very low-birthweight infants do not initially tolerate this level of glucose administration and have problems with hyperglycemia as well.

Hyperglycemia is commonly seen in very low-birthweight infants with RDS or those with evolving BPD. Their limited glucose tolerance may be due to decreased insulin production or decreased receptor response. Infants with significant respiratory or metabolic stress frequently have problems with hyperglycemia. The concurrent infusion of intravenous fat may also contribute to the problem of hyperglycemia.[17] Measures to correct hyperglycemia include lowering the glucose concentration and/or the rate of fluid administration, but both measures will limit the number of calories available to meet basal metabolic requirements and support growth.

Insulin, administered either intravenously or subcutaneously, is recommended by some researchers to improve glucose tolerance and increase caloric intake.[18-21] Other researchers have reported a diminished response to insulin in the premature.[22] Concerns about the use of insulin must be weighed against the known consequences of severe caloric deprivation in the premature.

Another area of concern regarding carbohydrate intake and chronic lung disease is the effect of high carbohydrate concentrations, used to supplement overall caloric intake, on respiratory physiology. Adults with chronic lung diseases were observed to have increased carbon dioxide levels while on high carbohydrate diets. Glucose metabolism increases carbon dioxide production and minute ventilation.[23,24] Carbon dioxide production is assessed by a method called indirect calorimetry, which measures oxygen consumption and carbon dioxide output with various diets. The breakdown of each nutrient is described as the ratio of carbon dioxide produced to oxygen consumed. Carbohydrate metabolism gives a respiratory quotient of 1.0 as compared to 0.8 for protein and 0.7 for fat. A respiratory quotient of 1.0 can potentially decrease respiratory reserve capacity and may be a negative factor in patients with respiratory insufficiency.[25,26] No studies to date have explored this measurement in infants with early BPD, but it may be prudent not to exceed 20 gm/kg/day of carbohydrate.

A balance between all the components of nutrition (protein, fat, and carbohydrate) is the goal when providing parenteral nutrition to the critically ill premature at risk for BPD during the acute phase of hospitalization. Meeting the caloric requirement for basal metabolic rate at rest is also a worthwhile goal during this time and will establish a foundation for better caloric and nutritional balance in the intermediate and chronic stages of BPD.

Complications of total parenteral nutrition are well documented and described in the literature. They include metabolic complications such as rickets, hepatic dysfunction from liver cholestasis, and septic complications. Thus, careful monitoring of appropriate metabolic and infection parameters is essential when providing either peripheral or total parenteral nutrition to neonates.[9,27]

**Vitamin and mineral status.** The role of vitamins is being explored in terms of the pathogenesis, prevention, and treatment of BPD. The results of the studies on vitamin E are inconclusive to date. One study reported a slightly lower incidence of BPD in infants who received vitamin E injections, an effect attributed to its antioxidant abilities.[28] Serum levels were 2–3 mg/dl (normal levels in adults are 1 mg/dl). A later study failed to show an effect on either incidence or severity of BPD in infants who received vitamin E and attained serum levels 3–5 mg/dl.[29] At the present time, vitamin E *sufficiency* appears to be the appropriate goal; by maintaining the vitamin E levels necessary for physiologic norms, the various organ systems dependent on this nutrient will receive what they require for baseline functioning. Sufficient levels of vitamin E have been attained using one vial of MVI Pediatric daily for term infants and 65 percent of a vial for prematures.[30]

Vitamin A (retinol) is another nutrient receiving scrutiny in the care of infants with BPD. The rationale for investigating the role of vitamin A in either preventing or treating BPD concerns its role in healing tissue. Vitamin A promotes epithelial repair after injury by stimulating differentiation of basal epithelial cells into the appropriate mucosal cell type. If vitamin A deficiency occurs, healing may be retarded and a squamous metaplasia can result. This metaplasia forms itself in the scar tissue in the tracheobronchial tree of the infant with BPD.[31]

Premature infants are deficient in vitamin A. They are born with lower liver reserves of vitamin A, low serum levels of vitamin A, and lower levels of retinol-binding protein than term infants.[32–34] Low vitamin A levels have been demonstrated in infants with BPD who were receiving intravenous vitamin A in concentrations of 400 IU/dl. (Normal concentrations of plasma vitamin A range from 25–90 μg/dl in adults.) This study indicated plasma levels of less than 20 μg/dl for up to 56 days after birth and less than 11 μg/dl for the first 28 days.[31] Another study confirmed these findings.[35]

A randomized, double-blind, controlled trial was conducted to determine the effect of vitamin A supplementation on morbidity associated with BPD in 40 very low-birthweight infants. Intramuscular vitamin A (retinol palmitate, 2,000 IU) was administered to 20 of the infants, 9 of whom developed BPD as compared to 17 of the control group. Of the infants given vitamin A, 75 percent achieved plasma levels greater than 20 μg/dl, and retinol-binding protein levels remained above baseline. The researchers speculate that vitamin A sufficiency promotes regenerative healing from lung injury.[36] It is important that studies be conducted to replicate these findings before clinical care recommendations are made.

An additional clinical note of interest arises from this study. The researchers chose the intramuscular route, in spite of the lack of muscle mass and other technical difficulties, because of studies indicating problems with intravenous delivery of vitamin A.[36] Although photodegradation of this nutrient has been described, the greatest loss of vitamin A is by adsorption into the plastic intravenous tubing.[37–39] Thus current methods of delivering intravenous vitamin A are unlikely to adequately provide this nutrient to infants who are relying on parenteral nutrition.

Providing adequate calcium and phosphorous for the infant in the early stage of illness of BPD also presents many challenges. Calcium is necessary for maintenance of cell membranes, neuromuscular activities, coagulation function, and bone mineralization. Phosphorous is a part of many metabolic reactions of organs and tissues; it is also involved with calcium metabolism in the process of bone accretion of these two minerals.

Premature infants have low stores of these minerals, which are deposited largely in the third trimester; diuretics have a potent effect on calcium and thereby on phosphorous status as well (Chapter 4). Thus the need for adequate delivery of these nutrients is higher in the population of very low-birth-weight infants who are developing BPD than in term or healthier premature infants. Providing 220–250 mg/kg of calcium and 120–150 mg/kg of phosphorous each day allows prematures to achieve optimal bone mineralization.[40]

There are problems in providing optimal concentrations of calcium and phosphorous in parenteral nutrition because of precipitation of calcium salts. Fluid restriction compounds the problem because higher mineral concentrations are necessary to supply daily requirements. It has been observed that the pH of the amino acid solution and the order in which the minerals are introduced during solution mixing can also lead to the development of precipitates.

The aforementioned vitamins and minerals are of special concern to those caring for infants who are at risk for developing BPD and who are receiving nutrition primarily through the parenteral route. It is important that all other nutrients also be carefully monitored.

## Vascular Access

Technical challenges in delivering intravenous nutrients to infants in the acute stage of illness are generally focused on issues of vascular access. Options include the use of umbilical arterial or venous catheters, peripheral IV lines, and central venous catheters.

Controversy still exists over using umbilical arterial or venous catheters to administer parenteral nutrition.[9] The major disadvantage of umbilical arterial lines is that their primary purpose is to provide a means of obtaining blood samples. Frequent breaks in the line for sampling increase the risk of infection in these compromised hosts, and many units have abandoned this practice as use of other routes has become more widespread. Umbilical venous lines used solely for the purpose of parenteral nutrition are utilized in some units. The catheter tip should be placed high in the inferior vena cava near the right atrium, especially if glucose concentrations greater than 12.5 percent are to be used. Risk of infection and prevalence of thrombus formation with the types of plastic catheters in most common use remain of concern.

Peripheral IV lines, either teflon catheters or steel needles, are still widely used. Major advantages are the low risk of infection and relative technical ease in placing catheters (up to a point). Protein concentrations up to 2 percent amino acids, carbohydrate concentrations up to 12.5 percent glucose, and intravenous fat concentrations of 10 or 20 percent have all been delivered safely via the peripheral venous route. However, as the infant progresses out of the acute and into the intermediate stage of illness, it is not really possible to provide adequate caloric intake *and* fluid restriction if peripheral parenteral solutions are the sole source of nutrition. Therefore, peripheral alimentation serves best in the early acute phase of illness, when basal metabolic needs alone are met, or as an adjunct to gavage feeding for the infant who is not getting enough calories from enteral nutrients.

Central venous catheters have many advantages in providing an optimal route for parenteral nutrition in the critically ill infant with evolving BPD. The central route allows for higher concentrations of amino acids and glucose and therefore allows for better fluid restriction. System stability means uninterrupted provision of nutrients (as compared to frequent IV starts using the peripheral route). The ability to infuse 3 percent or greater amino acids and 15 percent or greater dextrose solutions means higher, more consistent caloric intake. Another important advantage is the reduced trauma to the infant because the number of IV attempts is curtailed.

Disadvantages to the central venous route include an increased risk of infection, the potential of thrombus formation in large blood vessels, and technical difficulty placing lines in very small infants with tiny veins. Placing Broviac catheters or other surgically inserted lines usually requires general anesthesia and the loss of the vein as it is tied off for the procedure.

Another type of central venous catheter—the percutaneously placed silastic catheter—has recently become popular.[41,42] This very small, flexible catheter is inserted through a steel needle (19-gauge, scalp vein needle with extension tubing cut off. Newer sets being currently produced may have a "breakaway" needle.) The inserting needle is removed after placement of the catheter (usually 2 French silastic), and the catheter is then secured with a transparent dressing, such as OpSite or Tegaderm. Because of the delicate materials used to make these catheters, they cannot be sutured in place.

These silastic catheters may be placed in any vein that will accommodate the inserting needle. We have found the antecubital and scalp veins best suited for this procedure but have also used hand and jugular veins, and even the saphenous vein on occasion. Catheters are threaded into the superior vena cava at the junction of the right atrium or the inferior vena cava in the case of saphenous vein insertion. Tip location is confirmed by obtaining a chest x-ray using radiopaque contrast medium. Although many catheters are called "radiopaque," we have not found them suitable for initial determination of tip location.

Advantages to using the percutaneously placed catheters as compared to surgically placed lines include the following:

1. Because the vein is not ligated, there is no loss of the vessel; it may even be used at a later date for placement of another central line.
2. There is no need for general anesthesia or a trip to the operating room for placement.
3. Even in the lines placed in extremities, there is no need for long-term restraint on an arm board. (The flexible line tip is located in the large vessels in the infant's chest.)
4. Although there is a risk of infection, most units report relatively low rates of catheter-related sepsis with these lines (0.5–1 percent); our own experience with 128 catheters during a nine month period parallels this finding.[43]

Disadvantages of using these lines include the following:

1. There can be technical difficulties with insertion, such as lack of a vein suitable for cannulation or difficulty threading the line through the venous pathways into the large chest vessels.
2. The catheter cannot be used for blood withdrawal or administration because of the small lumen size.
3. Accidental dislodgement is a risk because the catheter cannot be sutured in place. (Most units using these catheters secure them with transparent dressing that is changed *only* if it starts to pull away from the skin.) These catheters also share with other central venous catheters the risks of pleural effusions, myocardial effusion, accidental severing of lines, and thrombus formation.

Care of central venous catheters in the neonate or young infant is a major nursing responsibility and should be described in detail by protocols established by each individual unit. Sample protocols available in Kerner's *Manual of Pediatric Parenteral Nutrition* may provide helpful information to units wishing to establish or expand their procedures.[9]

## Intermediate Stage

At this stage, acuity starts to subside, and chronicity becomes apparent. Many infants are still ventilator dependent but stable on moderate settings. Metabolic parameters are generally under control, and equipment such as chest tubes, arterial lines, and umbilical catheters are removed. There are usually attempts to begin enteral nutrition; in fact, the main goal during this stage is to establish enteral feeds as the major or sole source of nutritional intake. Superior nutritional status can be achieved only with an enteral diet.

Some units may elect to start enteral nutrition during the acute stage, feeling strongly that the superiority of enteral nutrition outweighs the risks

Other units feel that, although the benefits of enteral nutrition are obvious, risks such as necrotizing enterocolitis and factors such as poor intestinal motility make enteral feeding during the early stage of illness a less desirable or sometimes an impossible goal.

### Fluid and Energy Requirements

Fluid requirements during the intermediate stage are based on the same factors as those of the acute stage, but because certain problems are resolving, the tendency toward fluid imbalance may not be as strong. Insensible losses are lessened, for example, as the skin matures and better thermoregulation is achieved. Around the end of the second week of life, maintenance levels of fluid (100–150 cc/kg/day) are generally reached and well tolerated. As always, the fluid levels will need to be individualized according to the infant's medical status and other external factors. For example, the late appearance of a PDA may determine the need for a significant reduction of fluids for a particular infant.

Energy requirements (as indicated in Table 1) are similar to those in the acute phase, with a significant increase for the factors of growth and specific dynamic action. Specific dynamic action refers to the energy required to digest enteral feedings, so there is a range of caloric expenditures based on the amount of enteral feedings tolerated or achieved. Energy requirements for growth become central factors and are the second major component of caloric expenditures after the BMR. The total of 95–120 kcal/kg/day is almost double that of the acute stage and reflects the impact of growth on caloric intake.

Research into energy expenditures of infants with BPD as well as clinical findings of poor growth even at an enteral caloric intake of 120 kcal/kg day suggest that caloric needs during this stage may be even higher. Weinstein and Oh have demonstrated greater resting caloric expenditures in BPD infants due to increased resting oxygen consumption; they speculate the cause is higher respiratory rates and increased work of breathing.[44] If resting energy needs are not met, there certainly will be no calories available to support growth. More recent research indicates that infants with BPD who show poor growth experience increased oxygen consumption, whereas infants with BPD whose growth is adequate do not experience increased oxygen consumption.[45] Because the infants in this study were at six months corrected age, these findings may not be applicable to the intermediate stage of the disease. In general, it is probably safe to assume that there is an increase in oxygen consumption in most infants with BPD, and they may well need a caloric intake of 95–120 kcal/kg/day (depending on whether their nutrients are

**TABLE 2 ▪ Comparison of Energy and Protein Requirements in Parenteral and Enteral Nutrition**

| | PARENTERAL NUTRITION | ENTERAL NUTRITION |
|---|---|---|
| Energy | 70–120 kcal/kg/day | 115–130 kcal/kg/day |
| Protein | 2–3 gm/kg/day | 2.5–5 gm/kg/day |

provided enterally or parenterally) and possibly quite a bit higher to achieve adequate growth.

The differences in nutritional requirements of the parenteral versus the enteral route of delivery are marked (Table 2). One reason for these differences is that we assume 100 percent absorption and utilization from parenteral nutrition because there are no losses from digestion and stool. Another reason is that higher levels of protein delivered parenterally may overload the immature hepatic and renal system, resulting in BUN and ammonia elevations. However, a recent study has demonstrated the need for greater protein calories in neonates following surgery and suggests that this group may need above the recommended 3 gm/kg/day limit.[46] One of the clinical signs of protein malnutrition is the "flag sign," the appearance of white hair as the hair grows out. Infants with this sign have likely suffered a period of acute protein calorie malnutrition. We have observed this sign in some infants following surgery but also have seen it in some patients with prolonged, very acute courses of RDS progressing to BPD. Some adjustment of protein calories may therefore be recommended in certain circumstances, particularly if an extremely physiologically stressful hospital course is occurring.

### Nutritional Monitoring

Biochemical and metabolic factors requiring careful monitoring are similar to those of the acute phase. If prolonged parenteral nutrition is necessary, serum phosphorus, triglyceride, cholesterol, magnesium, SGOT, alkaline phosphatase, calcium, albumin, CBC, BUN, and creatinine are generally obtained weekly. Serum electrolyte determinations and glucose monitoring by Dextrostix or Chemstrips are ongoing; higher concentrations of glucose infusions are generally better tolerated by the infant at this stage. An advantage of using central lines to provide parenteral nutrition is that higher glucose and protein concentrations are able to be infused (dextrose concentrations up to 25 percent, amino acid solutions greater than 2 percent); thus appropriate caloric intake with fluid restriction is achieved.

**FIGURE 1 ▪ Computer printout indicates the fluid and calories received by an infant,** as well as the breakdown of nutrients (protein, fat, carbohydrate) received. This information, generated on a daily basis, helps determine nutritional needs for each individual patient. (Computer program information available at Children's Hospital, Oakland, California, Intensive Care Nursery)

```
-------CHILDRENS HOSPITAL MEDICAL CENTER-------
         East Bay Neonatology Associates
               Oakland, CA  96812

       ----Nutritional Analysis Program----
        Version 1.1 Copyright 1986, 1987

NUTRITION AND FLUID PROFILE FOR 05/25/89

Patient Name:                  PF#:
Weight: 1.520                  Weight Change From Yesterday: New

Fluids (cc/kg/24 hr):          126.3 Total
                               126.3 Free
                               0.0 (Blood Products + Meds + Flush)

Electrolytes (meq/kg/24 hr):   3.27 Sodium
                               3.69 Potassium

Output: Urine-    80.92 (cc/kg/24 hr) or    3.37 (cc/kg/hr)
        Total-    84.21 (cc/kg/24 hr) or    3.51 (cc/kg/hr)

Intake (calories/kg/24 hr) : 84.8    Total
                           : 37.2    IV
                           : 47.6    PO

Nutrients:   10.26 %PRO calories      1.50 grams of IV pro/kg/24 hr
             54.00 %CHO calories      1.28 grams of PO pro/kg/24 hr
             35.74 %FAT calories      0.66 grams of IV Fat/kg/24 hr
                                      2.63 grams of PO Fat/kg/24 hr
                                     12.83 grams of CHO/kg/24 hr

Ratio of Non-protein calories to Grams-protein:  27.9 to 1

                          ---------------
```

Nutritional calculations necessary on a daily basis for these patients in the intermediate stage of illness include determinations of calories and fluids (kg/day) and sodium and potassium (mEq/kg/day). It is also extremely useful to calculate grams of protein, fat, and carbohydrate received per kilogram each day and to have a breakdown of the percentage of these nutrients that comprise the total intake. These figures can guide the clinician in selecting which nutrients may safely be increased to improve overall caloric intake and provide better balanced nutrition. Figure 1 shows a sample of a computer printout that is generated daily on each patient in our unit, providing this information in an efficient and accurate fashion.

Because growth is the major goal during this and all subsequent stages of

**FIGURE 2 ■ Physiologic and Anatomic Handicaps of the GI Tract in Premature Infants**

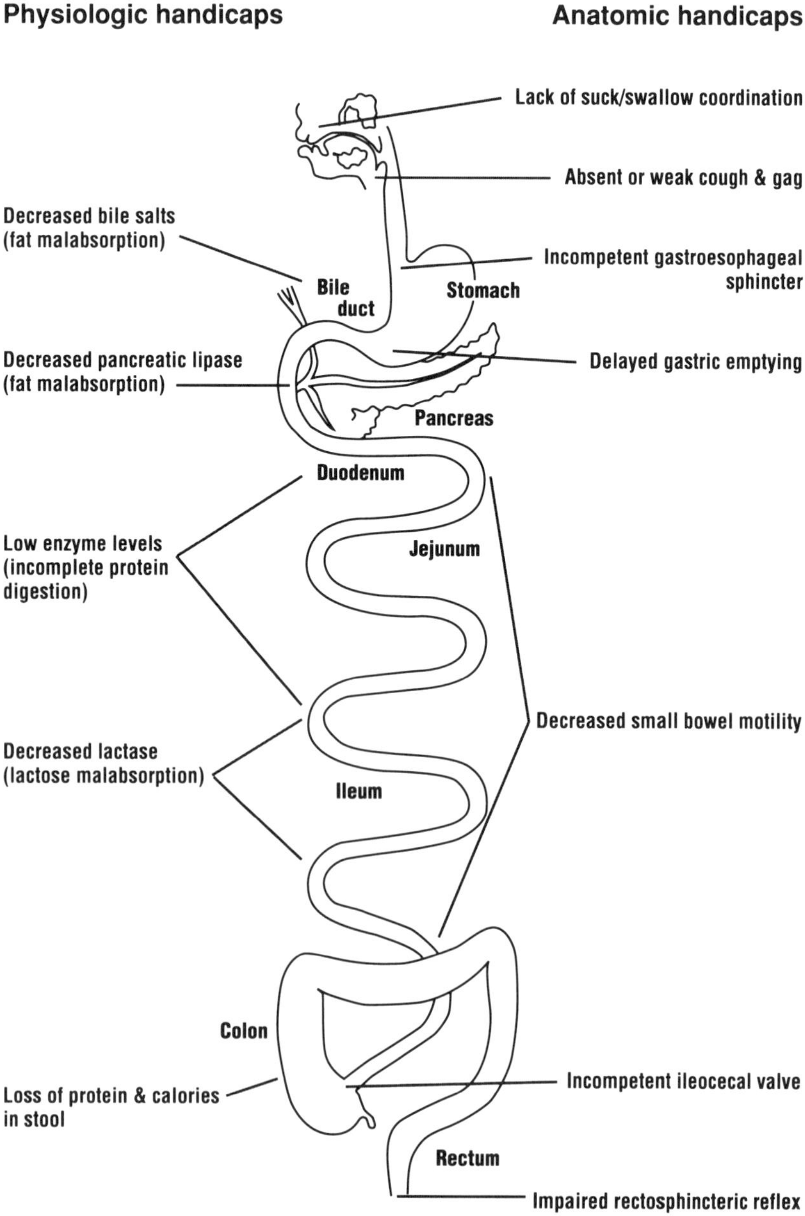

illness, careful attention to growth parameters will help in assessing the adequacy of the energy and protein intake being provided. Typically, weight is measured daily, length and head circumference, weekly. Measurements should be plotted on an appropriate growth chart. A variety of charts are available, including the Babson growth chart. Many infants will display growth patterns that differ from intrauterine growth. However, as each infant establishes an upward trend of growth on his own curve, there is hope that future growth patterns may indicate some degree of "catch-up" growth.

### Enteral Nutrition

Establishing enteral feedings at the level necessary to deliver nutrients adequate to support growth is the major goal and challenge of this intermediate stage. Both physiologic and anatomic handicaps of the premature infant's gastrointestinal tract lead to difficulties in establishing enteral feedings (Figure 2). The overall motility of the small bowel is impaired in the premature infant, and particularly in certain infants with BPD who fail to propel their formula through their gastrointestinal tract and regularly have gastric residuals and abdominal distention.[47] Attempts to prevent necrotizing enterocolitis in this high-risk group also result in numerous unsuccessful starts and stops on the road to establishing enteral nutrition for many infants.

The decision as to the best tolerated method for providing feedings is based not only on the infant's medical status and size; it also tends to reflect the firmly held nutritional views of the unit. For example, a premature infant on generous ventilator settings may benefit from a continuous nasogastric infusion feeding, as opposed to a bolus gavage feeding, to prevent stomach expansion and increased pressure on the diaphragm with resulting respiratory compromise.[48] For many infants, however, a bolus-type gavage feeding using a nasogastric or orogastric tube is the preferred method.

There are several advantages to the bolus or intermittent gavage method. If breast milk is used, there is less separation of fat and liquid than with a continuous slow infusion.[49] Nutrients such as calcium and phosphorous may also be lost when formulas are infused.[50] For an infant with slightly delayed gastric emptying, bolusing a larger volume may help stimulate gastric motility and prevent problems with residuals. Nonnutritive sucking on a pacifier may also stimulate motility and has the added advantage of helping the infant associate the sensation of feeding with sucking. Bolus, or intermittent, gavage feeds can be given as often as every hour for infants with small stomach capacity or problems with reflux or residuals; however, three-hour feeding intervals are more commonly used.

**TABLE 3 ■ Comparison of Three Tube Feeding Methods**

| METHOD | ADVANTAGES | DISADVANTAGES |
|---|---|---|
| Bolus (gavage) | 1. Better delivery of nutrients: less separation of fat in breastmilk, more calcium and phosphorus delivered in premature formulas<br>2. Stimulates gastric emptying<br>3. Feelings of fullness and emptiness may establish hunger/satiation cycle for later feeding motivation<br>4. Less concern about bacterial overgrowth in breast milk | 1. Pressure on diaphragm will decrease lung expansion when the stomach is full<br>2. Potential increased risk of aspiration, vomiting, and reflux because the stomach becomes fuller |
| Continuous Nasogastric drip | 1. Less pressure on the diaphragm, more room for lung expansion<br>2. Decreased risk of aspiration, vomiting, and reflux because the stomach is never completely "full" | 1. Impaired delivery of nutrients: fat in breast milk separates, calcium and phosphorus settle out in premature formulas<br>2. Potential for bacterial overgrowth, especially if breast milk is used<br>3. More expensive: new tubing every 8 hours<br>4. Does not allow for feelings of hunger/satiation to be established |
| Transpyloric (nasoduodenal, nasojejunal) | 1. Risks of aspiration, vomiting, and reflux virtually removed<br>2. Delayed gastric emptying will no longer limit feeding tolerance, because the stomach is bypassed<br>3. Decreased pressure on the diaphragm allows better lung expansion | 1. Potential for malabsorption if tube slips too far into the jejunum<br>2. Impaired delivery of nutrients, especially fat in breast milk, calcium and phosphorous in premature formula<br>3. Risk of perforation with certain types of tubes<br>4. Technical difficulties of passing the tube into the small bowel, delays in feeding if tube becomes dislodged<br>5. Benefit of gastric HCl on digestive process is eliminated |

Aspiration is a very real concern in the population of premature and term infants likely to develop BPD, particularly if they are fed via the gavage route while intubated. Between 60 and 80 percent of infants studied in one center showed evidence of pulmonary aspiration of dye placed on their tongue, a finding that suggests that if milk reaches the oral cavity (from vomiting or reflux), there is a high likelihood of aspiration.[51]

Nursing measures to prevent aspiration in intubated infants on gavage feedings include facilitating gastric emptying by prone or right-side-down positioning, elevating the head of the bed to a 30° angle, and promoting better motility by encouraging nonnutritive sucking and establishing appropriate stooling patterns.

Transpyloric feedings have been suggested for infants with severe reflux who are at high risk for aspiration. We have also used this method in infants with very poor gastric emptying who have failed numerous attempts to establish feeding by either bolus or continuous infusion techniques. Transpyloric feedings (nasoduodenal or nasojejunal) decrease the chance of vomiting, aspiration, and reflux by bypassing the stomach and emptying the milk directly into the small intestine; the pyloric sphincter of the stomach prevents reflux of milk back into the stomach. Disadvantages of this method include the following: (1) possible malabsorption, especially if the tube slips too far down into the jejunum, thereby preventing the milk from mixing with pancreatic enzymes; (2) perforation, especially with stiffer tubes; (3) difficulty in placing and keeping the tube in the correct position; and (4) the necessity of feeding continuously (rather than bolus) because the intestine, unlike the stomach, cannot function as a reservoir.[52] Table 3 summarizes the advantages and disadvantages of bolus, continuous drip, and transpyloric feeding methods.

Choice of milk is variable and not entirely determined by feeding method. Breast milk is frequently used as an initial feeding, because many mothers try to pump, at least for a while, and have frozen milk available for initial feedings. A number of reasons make it difficult to maintain lactation—extremely premature birth, high stress level for mother, fatigue at frequent pumping. Many mothers become overwhelmed at the prospect of pumping for the many months that their infant will remain ventilator dependent. We encourage mothers and assist them in their pumping efforts, but we feel it necessary to help them realistically evaluate how they will maintain lactation for the weeks or months ahead. If breast milk is used, supplementation with some type of fortifier will probably be necessary in order to provide higher caloric density and higher protein intake and improve mineral intake because the infant with BPD has greater requirements for these nutrients.

If breast milk is not available or if supplies are inadequate, the formulas designed for premature infants provide an excellent digestible source of the additional nutrients required by the infant with BPD. These formulas, with their high vitamin and calcium supplements, are ideally suited for the BPD infant; if other formulas are used, it is necessary to supplement with additional vitamins and minerals, which add to the osmotic load in the gastrointestinal tract.

Initially, a 20 kcal/oz formula is used, and some units may dilute this to half strength in an effort to stimulate the intestinal villi without stressing them with a full osmotic load. A slow, cautious approach follows, with increases in volume alternating with increases in strength until the infant is receiving 120 kcal/kg/day and exhibiting appropriate growth. (Some infants may require even higher caloric intake to achieve growth.) Careful monitoring of stools, abdominal girth, residuals, and vomiting patterns is basic to the care of these infants. Growth need not be compromised while enteral feeds are being established if they are supplemented with parenteral nutrients.

## Chronic Stage

This stage begins as the infant with BPD becomes more stable physiologically, perhaps weans from the ventilator, and is being cared for with hood, tent, cannula, or tracheostomy oxygen supplements. The goals of this stage, from a nutritional standpoint, include establishing fluid hemostasis with or without diuretics, providing optimal caloric intake to promote growth in all parameters, and beginning oral or nipple feedings in preparation for home care.

### Fluid and Energy Requirements

An infant's fluid status can be as frustrating to manage during this stage as it was during the acute phase of the illness. Most often the problem lies with fluid excesses and the need to restrict fluid while still providing optimal calories. The use of diuretics is now widespread, allowing the use of higher fluid intake to some extent. A typical fluid restriction required by a BPD infant is 130–150 cc/kg/day; for some infants, however, this may be too much fluid even with diuretics, and they may need to be restricted to less than 130 cc/kg/day.

Energy requirements for the chronic stage of illness are determined by the same components as those in the intermediate stage (Table 1). The total number of calories (120–130 kcal/kg/day) is slightly higher, however, because of the influence of increased activity, regulation of body temperature outside the incubator or warming table, and increased specific dynamic action as enteral feedings become the sole source of calories. Recent research has demonstrated higher metabolic rates due to elevated oxygen consumption in infants of six months corrected age with growth failure (height and weight at less than the tenth percentile) who had BPD. Infants with BPD who showed adequate growth did not exhibit these higher rates of oxygen consumption and likely did not need higher caloric intakes.[45] A further study has demonstrated that neither a lower caloric intake nor fecal loss of nutrients was responsible for poorer growth.[53] The mystery of poor growth in certain BPD infants remains, but perhaps increased need for certain nutrients, such as protein, plays a significant role.

We have seen patients who exhibit adequate growth with relatively low caloric intakes, as well as those requiring in excess of 130 kcal/kg/day. Both extremes indicate the individual differences in metabolic rates inherent in infants with BPD. Indirect calorimetry would provide a method to determine the *individual* infant's energy needs so that a nutritional plan could be tailor-made for each patient. This, however, remains a research tool, and clinicians must continue to struggle along, looking at intake, weight, and growth curves to determine the adequacy of nutritional management.

Parameters for monitoring nutritional status during this stage are basically the same as those in the intermediate stage. Weekly measurements of length and head circumference are plotted on an appropriate growth chart; weight is obtained daily or every other day and plotted on the chart every week. Frequently, infants do not follow the established growth curves. It is more important to determine if the infant has established a pattern of growth reflected in his own curve and then to investigate deviations from this curve than to be overly concerned about where he fits on the established curve. Figure 3 shows the growth curve of an infant with BPD who has established a growth pattern below that of the norms but with a definite upward trend.

Laboratory monitoring during this stage is greatly reduced, because the infant is no longer on parenteral nutrition. Occasional electrolyte determinations are necessary for the infant receiving diuretics. Hemoglobin, hematocrit, and reticulocyte counts are obtained in order to ensure that the levels are optimal for improving oxygen-carrying capacity and to evaluate if the infant is producing red blood cells. Other monitoring may include an assessment of bone mineralization via x-ray examination and serum determination of micronutrients including alkaline phosphatase, calcium and phosphorous to determine if deficiencies exist.

Bone demineralization, hypophosphatemia, and rickets are frequently encountered in infants with BPD. Causes of these conditions include prematurity and low calcium stores, parenteral nutrition and inadequate delivery of calcium and phosphorous, vitamin D deficiency, and use of unsupplemented

**FIGURE 3 ■ Babson growth chart shows the growth of a three month old infant with BPD.** Although he is below the tenth percentile, his growth shows that he has established an appropriate curve as he begins to gain weight and length.

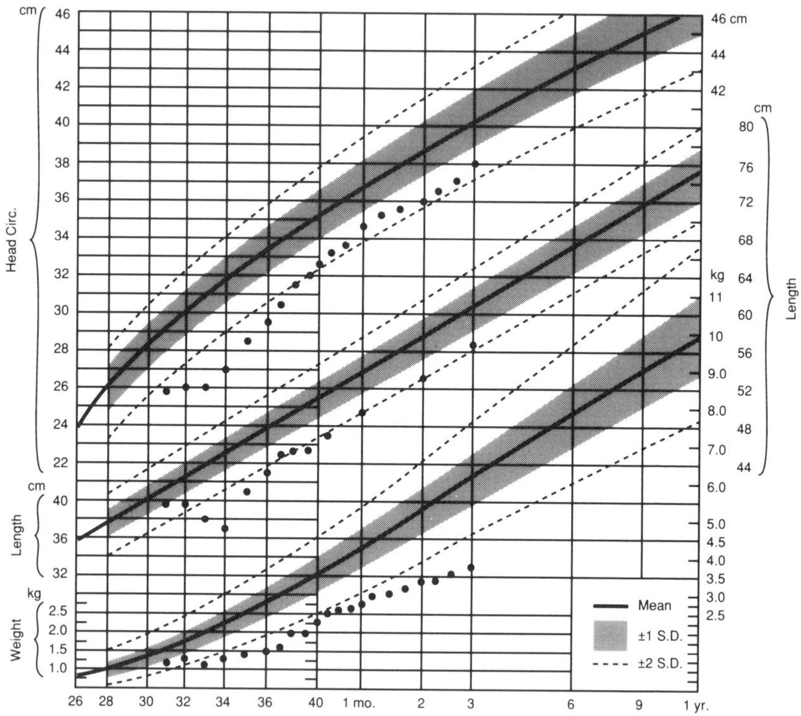


From: Babson SG, and Benda GI: Growth graphs for the clinical assessment of infants of varying gestational ages, Journal of Pediatrics 89, 1976, p. 814.

human milk or formulas not designed for the premature infant. Infants with bone demineralization may suffer pathologic fractures and be in considerable discomfort. Treatment for severe cases includes vitamin D supplementation (use of fortifiers in breastmilk), calcium and phosphorous supplementation, or prolonged use of premature formulas to supply the extra amounts of appropriate micronutrients the infant requires.[54,55]

## Gastroesophageal Reflux

Passage of gastric contents into the esophagus, called gastroesophageal reflux (GER), is a common finding among newborns and is even more frequently found among premature infants. Infants with GER have small to large amounts of emesis that seem to just roll out of their mouths following feedings, as opposed to the projectile vomiting seen with pyloric stenosis, increased intracranial pressure, or gastroenteritis. Infants with pulmonary diseases such as asthma, chronic bronchitis, recurrent pneumonias, and BPD have a high incidence of GER.[56,57]

Gastroesophageal reflux is considered serious or pathologic if there is evidence of failure to thrive in spite of adequate intake, aspiration and pneumonia from refluxed contents, or esophagitis from the acidic nature of the refluxed gastric materials.[58] Some infants may also experience bradycardia or airway compromise during episodes of GER resulting from vagal stimulation or airway compression.[59,60]

When an infant with BPD has a problem with frequent emesis, it may be helpful to determine if GER is a factor. Diagnostic methods currently being used include upper GI series with barium, esophagoscopy, esophageal biopsy, pH probe monitoring of the esophagus, esophageal pressure manometry, radionuclide study, and sleep studies.[61]

Once the diagnosis of GER is confirmed and its negative consequences (such as failure to thrive or recurrent pneumonia) are determined, various therapies are attempted. Supportive nursing care measures involving positioning and feeding are often instituted. Current recommendations for optimal positions during feeding include (1) prone position rather than sitting upright in an infant seat, (2) prone position with the head elevated to a 30–45° angle using a harness to keep the baby from sliding down, and (3) prone position with the use of a "slant board," which enables movement of the infant's arms and supports the infant's buttocks to prevent sliding off.[58,62,63]

Feedings thickened with infant cereal flakes to provide a heavier material that is less likely to reflux up the esophagus are often used for the infant with GER. Two recent studies of the efficacy of this approach showed differing results. One found that, although thickened feedings actually delayed gastric emptying, this did not worsen GER. In fact, favorable effects were seen, including increased caloric content with the cereal-thickened feedings, decreased emesis, decreased crying time, and increased sleep time after feedings.[64] The other study found no difference in reflux after thickened feedings. This study did not look at the effect of head-up positioning in addition to thickening, which is the most common position used.[65] Although research has not proven the efficacy of this technique to reduce GER in the infant with BPD, many clinicians maintain these measures in their arsenal of noninvasive strategies to treat GER.[66]

Other feeding strategies sometimes employed for infants with severe GER include frequent, small-volume gavage feedings (every one to two hours), continuous nasogastric feedings (to decrease milk volume in the stomach at any given time), and the transpyloric feeding route.[56] These methods are effective on a short-term basis to promote weight gain and diminish pulmonary complications, but they are not optimal for long-term and home care in most cases because of their numerous technical disadvantages.

Medication has also been used with varying success in the treatment of GER. Metoclopramide (Reglan) may be helpful if delayed gastric emptying is a component of the reflux problem. Its action includes hastening gastric emptying, improving the tone of the upper gastrointestinal tract, and reducing nausea.[67] Onset of action is approximately 30–60 minutes after oral administration; the usual dose is 0.01–0.15 mg/kg/day, given in three to four divided doses before feedings. Adverse reactions include restlessness, drowsiness, and fatigue.

A recent study of the efficacy of metoclopramide for treatment of GER indicates it may actually exacerbate the symptoms of GER in some infants.[68] Another drug used to treat GER is bethanecol; because one of the side effects of this drug is bronchospasm, it is generally not used in infants with BPD.

If a particular infant does not receive any relief of GER symptoms in spite of the above therapies and if failure to thrive, frequent pneumonias, apnea, or esophagitis continues, surgical intervention may be considered. The most common procedure employed to correct GER is the Nissen fundoplication. In this procedure, the stomach is used to "wrap" the distal esophagus and stabilize the cardiac sphincter, creating at this junction a partial closure that prevents gastric contents from re-entering the esophagus. The surgery is fairly complex, requiring general anesthesia and an experienced surgeon to ensure success.[61]

Problems following this procedure generally result from a "too-tight wrap" clinically manifested as gas bloat, inability to vomit, dysphagia, poor appetite due to early satiety, and the need for gastric decompression via nasogastric or gastrostomy tube. Another complication associated with the procedure is small bowel obstruction secondary to adhesions.[69]

The treatments available for GER remain varied and to some extent controversial. It is clear, however, that many infants with BPD will continue to be plagued with this condition and that a spectrum of therapies based on individual needs and responses will be employed.

## Oral Feedings

Once an infant can tolerate all or most of the caloric intake needed for appropriate growth by enteral feedings (either gavage or continuous nasogastric), introducing oral or nipple feedings becomes the next goal. Before attempting this phase, the infant's readiness and maturity are assessed, and respiratory stability must be attained.

Most premature infants exhibit readiness for nipple feedings by 34 weeks gestation. Readiness is indicated by maturation of the sucking reflex and pattern, the strength of sucking, and the ability to coordinate the suck-swallow-breathe sequence as a bolus of milk passes over the pharynx while the epiglottis temporarily closes. Coordination of suck and swallow is largely determined by the cranial oropharyngeal nerves.[70]

Respiratory disease interferes in several ways with the readiness and ability to attempt oral feedings. The prolonged need for mechanical ventilation prevents many infants from attempting their first oral feeding until well beyond 40 weeks postconception. There may be a critical period in the progression of reflexive feeding behavior to learned feeding actions that is missed in some BPD infants who remain intubated for months past their due dates. In addition, the oral feeding ability of the infant with chronic pulmonary disease is compromised by fatigue (from increased work of breathing), low energy reserves or tolerance for activity, difficulty coordinating suck-swallow-breathe sequence with respiratory rates in the range of 60–100/minute, and feeding-associated hypoxia.[71,72]

The instrumentation used to treat the BPD infant may also have negative consequences. Swallowing dysfunction, which may resemble bulbar paralysis, has been described following tracheostomy.[73] The prolonged effects of endotracheal intubation and noxious oral stimulation from suctioning may have a negative effect on later feeding behavior. In addition, chronic respiratory disease necessitates long-term hospitalization and prevents the normal development of maternal-infant attachment in which feeding is the cornerstone.

### Feeding Dysfunction

The challenge of establishing oral feedings in the BPD infant is complex. Because there are a multitude of potential causes of feeding dysfunction or disability, it is important to try to determine the cause of feeding difficulty before determining a course of action. This is a relatively new area of exploration in the care of infants. Three of the causes of feeding dysfunction that have been identified to date are lack of coordination, oral-motor dysfunction, and feeding resistance.

**Lack of coordination (the "disorganized" feeder).** The disorganized feeder is generally a premature infant who is ready to attempt feedings around 40 weeks or shortly thereafter. Chapter 6 provides an excellent overview of the process of feeding infants like this and suggests numerous feeding strategies. Among the suggestions are (1) preparing the infant by helping him attain an optimal behavioral state before feedings and (2) pacing the feeding with appropriate pauses based on the infant's cues and indications of vital sign or respiratory instability. Using nipples with a flow appropriate to the infant's ability to swallow is also important, as is warming the milk to promote a more positive tactile experience. Eliminating competing forms of stimulation, such as talking to the infant or making eye contact, can also be helpful.

These infants usually progress best if feedings are introduced slowly, starting with one per day, moving to one per shift, and gradually to every other feeding. Some infants respond better to a set volume of milk per shift, rather than a set volume for each feeding: This allows them to consume smaller volumes more frequently and permits feeding times to be based on their readiness and interest. It is essential to monitor the infant's individual physiologic response to feeding; this helps the caretaker assess the need to either increase supplemental oxygen or stop the feeding.

**Oral-motor dysfunction.** This type of feeding disorder is seen in infants with a neurologically mediated sucking and/or swallowing problem. Feeding difficulties in this group of infants may represent cranial nerve abnormalities, such as bulbar palsy, or generalized central nervous system abnormalities, such as hypoxic encephalopathy, hydrocephaly, microcephaly, or cerebral palsy. A recent pilot study differentiated the sucking patterns seen in infants with disorganized feeding problems (discussed above) from those with oral-motor dysfunction. Deviant jaw function and generalized hypotonia were observed in the dysfunction group.[74] Professionals skilled in assessing lip, tongue, and mouth movements may be needed to make this differentiation.

Special feeding teams have been developed in some pediatric centers to help children with multiple feeding problems. Team members include the primary nurse or caretaker, physician, nutritionist, physical therapist, occupational therapist, and speech pathologist. One such program, used to establish oral feedings in children after long-term gastrostomy feedings, consists of the following elements:

- Initial evaluation to rule out inadequate swallowing and gastroesophageal reflux and to determine developmental readiness for behavior modification techniques (need to be functioning at a five-month level)
- Determination of the most appropriate setting for success, inpatient versus outpatient (It might be expected that the infant's mother would have the most success, but many parents find the program too difficult to carry out at home.)

- Preparation—tube feedings are placed on a schedule similar to normal eating and snacking times, adequate caloric intake levels are determined, and oral-motor exercises and desensitization are carried out
- Treatment using behavior modification techniques with the occupational therapist acting as a "model" for caretakers[75]

**Feeding resistance.** This type of feeding disorder may be encountered in chronically ill hospitalized infants with initial disorganized or dysfunctional feeding patterns. These early abnormal patterns, along with long-term use of tube feedings or total parenteral nutrition that bypasses normal feeding pathways and prolonged hospitalization with multiple caretakers, can lead to feeding resistance. The pattern of resistance, once established, can take months to unravel because these infants are frequently quite persistent and usually at a developmental stage when control and mastery of some aspect of their environment is important. The feeding experience is one of the few areas in which they can exert their control, usually with great impact on their frustrated parent or nurse.

We have seen resistance to feeding in infants with BPD as well as in infants with a surgical condition or other chronic illnesses. The following behaviors are seen: turning the head when approached with a rubber nipple or pacifier, thrusting out the tongue when the nipple enters the mouth, rumination or retching when the liquid enters the mouth or pharynx, falling asleep when feeding is attempted. Some infants have an overall aversion to all oral stimulation, including nonnutritive sucking on fingers or pacifiers; others enjoy nonnutritive sucking but instantly know the difference when liquid follows the nipple.

The following approach to overcoming feeding resistance, which was directed and largely carried out by the primary nurse, has been described in case reports:

- Desensitize the facial area around the mouth and cheeks with gentle stroking of the cheek and lips, coupled with positive social interaction and reinforcement
- When the facial area is desensitized, attempt to introduce fingers or objects into the infant's mouth
- Decrease invasive oral procedures as much as possible, and clearly separate them in time and setting from positive oral stimulation periods
- Associate oral stimulation during feeding with social interaction[76,77]

Before any such program is implemented, it is necessary to clearly identify any other components of the feeding resistance, such as airway obstruction, neurologic abnormalities, or active infection. Other complicating factors such as oral candida infections, electrolyte disturbances, hyperammonemia, acidosis, vitamin deficiency, or zinc deficiency can contribute to anorexia or suck and swallow aberrations and should be investigated as well.[78,79]

### Feeding Strategies

A variety of health professionals including nurses, physical therapists, occupational therapists, infant developmental specialists, speech pathologists, nutritionists, gastroenterologists, parents, and even volunteers have been involved in implementing various feeding plans.

**Prevention.** Early interventions may reduce some of the feeding pathology seen in the intensive care nursery. The developmental care plan instituted early in the course of care for the infant at risk for BPD should promote better positioning by encouraging flexed posture in either side lying or prone and a head position that avoids constant neck extension. Hand-to-mouth activity is facilitated, under supervision, as much as possible when the infant indicates readiness. Positive stimulation is provided to the cheeks and lips (when retaping the endotracheal tube, for example) with firm, gentle massage. The pacifier or caretaker's finger (dipped in 10 percent glucose water solution if the infant prefers) is offered for nonnutritive sucking, especially during tube feedings. When they are stable enough, these infants are held during feedings to condition them to a more normal feeding regime.

By using these measures, we may be better able to help infants associate the feeling of fullness with holding and sucking activity. If any intervention elicits negative response from the infant, it is essential to cease and use a less noxious intervention until the infant signals readiness to move on.

**Breastfeeding.** Some infants in our experience have successfully breastfed after prolonged ventilation for BPD and the need for long-term supplemental oxygen therapy. Recent research indicates that breastfeeding may be somewhat less physiologically stressful than bottle feeding for healthy premature infants, as evidenced by more stable heart rate, respiratory rate, temperature, and $TcPO_2$ readings.[80,81] Although this work has not yet been replicated on infants with BPD, we have found breastfeeding beneficial for several infants in our practice. Indicators for success seem to involve (1) a good milk supply and well-established let-down reflex (no small accomplishment for mothers who have been pumping for months), (2) support for the mother during feeding, with a nurse observing the infant's vital signs and oxygenation status, (3) supplemental oxygen when indicated using a nasal cannula directly under the infant's nares, and (4) use of a supplemental nursing system (SNS-Medela or Lact-Aid nurser) when the milk supply is not adequate or a supplement is needed to boost the caloric density or mineral status of the breast milk.

Investigators have clearly outlined some maneuvers to facilitate appropriate sucking techniques for the breastfed infant, including oral stimulation with the finger prior to feeding and methods to assess tongue and lip actions while feeding.[82] In addition, offering the breast during the first few feedings and as much as possible after the initial experience seems to better train the infant to the appropriate sucking pattern and helps avoid nipple confusion. Although breastfeeding has not been a realistic goal for all our BPD infants, it can work well for some and should be attempted.

**Combined tube and nipple feedings**. When an infant starts to take 25–30 percent of his feedings by nipple, it is helpful to establish a feeding regimen that encourages the positive rewards of nipple feeding without tiring the infant or frustrating the caretaker. We have used the following two approaches successfully:

1. Using a polyurethane feeding tube (6 French) passed nasally and left in place. This type of plastic does not harden and can be left in place for up to 30 days. This reduces the need to pass a new nasogastric tube daily and results in less negative oral stimulation. Feedings can be partially nippled and the remainder gavaged to reach the full volume.

   An alternative method allows the infant to nipple feed as much milk as tolerated for a six to eight hour period, after which the amount of formula needed to make an appropriate caloric intake can be added. The small sized tube generally does not compromise respiration. The impact of the indwelling tube on feeding ability should be assessed; some infants may benefit by having the tube removed during the nipple feeding period and reinserted only when supplemental gavage feeding is required.
2. Establishing a period of time for ad lib nipple feedings (such as 7 am to 7 pm, or 6 am to 10 pm) to allow the infant to self-regulate volume and frequency of feeding. The infant is then gavage fed during the remainder of the day (or continuously fed by drip method) to a prescribed volume. As the infant's intake increases, the amount of supplemented feeding is reduced. We have had success with this method, which we attribute to the infant's self-regulation of feeding and also to the impact of hunger.

   A feeding flow sheet is a useful tool in determining a more consistent nippling approach. Although some infants might be able to respond to different feeding styles and techniques, others may become confused, just as some infants become confused when they are on a combined breast and bottle feeding regimen.

**Increasing caloric density of formula.** Infants who require extra calories to grow yet also need fluid restriction to reduce lung water may require formula with a caloric density well above 20 kcal/oz. A 24 kcal/oz formula is readily available and utilized widely in most intensive care nurseries, both in premature preparations and in standard formulas. Higher caloric density may also be needed if fluid homeostasis is even more delicate or if a given infant is simply unable to take adequate volumes by mouth in spite of well-established feeding behaviors.

Caloric density of formula can be increased using carbohydrate in the form of glucose polymers (powdered provides 8 kcal/teaspoon, liquid 2 kcal/cc) and fat in the form of MCT oil (8.3 kcal/gm or 7.7 kcal/cc) or safflower oil (9 kcal/gm or 8.4 kcal/cc). Carbohydrate is generally well tolerated but may result in diarrhea in some infants. An additional concern is that the infant may gain fat but not muscle mass, so additional protein may be necessary to achieve better growth of muscle.[83] Fat supplementation has resulted in fatty stools for some of our patients, and there is some evidence that fat can delay gastric emptying and decrease appetite.[84,85] It is important also to maintain an adequate percentage of calories from protein (8–10 percent) when increasing the caloric density with nonprotein supplements.

Another approach is simply to make an overall higher density formula by using a standard powdered formula and adding less water. We have used this technique to achieve a caloric density as high as 28–30 kcal/oz. Concentrating formulas does result in increased osmolarity, but many infants will tolerate this increase if it is gradually advanced and do well with formulas of 28–30 kcal/oz. Some centers report using carbohydrate—and fat—supplemented formulas up to 32–45 kcal/oz (1.1–1.5 kcal/cc); we have not had experience with this range of caloric density and generally have seen adequate growth at lower densities.

**Introducing solid foods.** At about three to four months corrected age, many infants exhibit readiness for solid food delivered by a spoon. Readiness may come somewhat later in the infant with BPD because of the infant's instability and developmental delay due to neurologic conditions or environmental deprivation. Cereals may have already been introduced in an effort to decrease gastroesophageal reflux.

The major reason for introducing solids is *not* to provide nutritional enhancement: It is to promote oral-motor skills and developmental activities necessary for later feeding, eating, and language skills. Spoon feeding should be introduced under the guidance of a developmental program so that readiness and acceptance can be adequately assessed before moving on to the next step. Solid food, in general, lacks the nutritional completeness and caloric density of supplemented formulas. If infants take increased amounts of certain solids, such as fruit, they may replace their usual intake of milk and reduce their protein intake. Foods such as high-protein cereal, fruit-flavored yogurt, pudding, sweet potatoes, or ice cream are good choices because they are higher in calories, lower in fluid, and higher in protein than many other foods. Also, many infants may find these foods more appealing during the early initiation of solid foods.[86] Later, meat should be added because of its protein content. Handbooks of nutrient values of solids should be obtained from the various baby food companies and consulted when designing a diet for the BPD infant.[87]

Liquids by cup are not initially handled as easily as solids and take longer to establish. We have seen some infants who were able to take solid foods by spoon without ever mastering nipple feedings. This type of progression is not optimal because the tongue and jaw movements that nippling stimulates are used later during speech acquisition. However, some infants are unable to ever establish nipple feedings and probably utilize other strategies to compensate for the lack of normal oral developmental process.

### Gastrostomy Feedings

Certain circumstances necessitate the insertion of a gastrostomy tube. Infants who require a fundoplication for treatment of gastroesophageal reflux generally have a gastrostomy tube placed because this is the only way feedings or air can be expelled following the procedure. [61] Gastrostomy is also considered for infants who have delayed oral feeding abilities, such as a severe dysfunctional feeding pattern or feeding resistance. Infants with specific sucking and swallowing disorders that place them at high risk for aspiration are also candidates for gastrostomy tube placement.[88] Generally, we consider gastrostomy tube placement if, at or near the time of discharge, an infant is taking less than 50 percent of his intake orally, and it is assessed that the ability to increase this amount substantially will take months.

Some infants may tolerate the use of an indwelling polyurethane nasogastric feeding tube to supplement oral intake. However, there are several drawbacks to this approach such as risk of aspiration, influence of the tube on nippling progress, and worsening GER symptoms due to the presence of the tube. The decision to place a gastrostomy tube or use long-term nasogastric feeding tubes is made for each individual infant after careful evaluation.

A standard gastrostomy tube is placed if the initial purpose of the tube is gastric decompression (as after a fundoplication). If the tube is placed expressly for feeding purposes or maintained after decompression is no longer the key issue, a gastrostomy feeding button may have some advantages. The

**FIGURE 4 ■ The gastrostomy feeding button has several advantages:** easier skin care, less bulky, infant cannot remove it, no chance that the tube can slip into the duodenum.

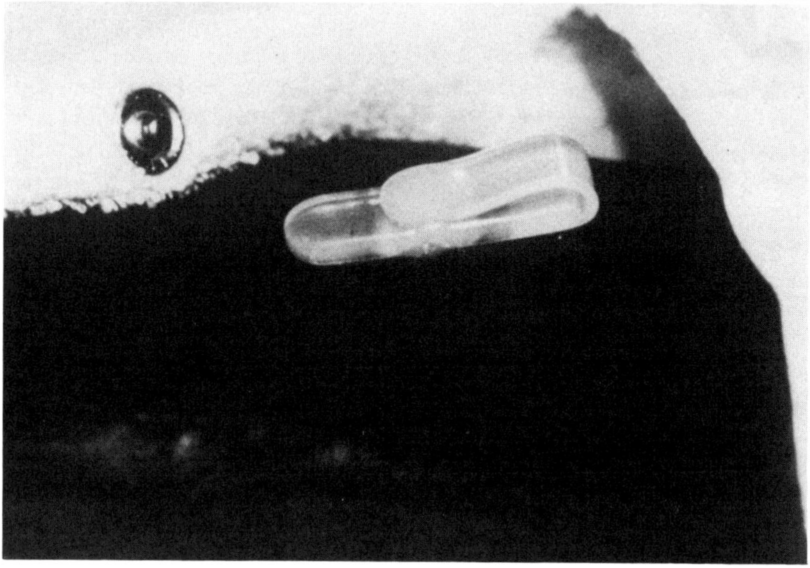

button is a small, flexible device made of silicon about an inch long. The end inserted into the stomach has a mushroom-shaped dome with a one-way valve that allows the feeding to enter and prevents stomach contents from coming back out. The end that is at skin level has two plastic wings that hold it onto the infant and a plastic "plug" to close the button after the feeding (see Figure 4).

Advantages and disadvantages of the button are well described in a recent article.[89] The major advantage we have observed is the more acceptable appearance and improved skin condition at the stoma site with the feeding button as compared with conventional gastrostomy tubes. In addition, dislodgment by the patient is almost impossible, and there is a decreased risk of migration and intestinal obstruction as compared with standard gastrostomy tubes, which can migrate into the duodenum despite careful efforts to secure them properly. Drawbacks to the button include difficulty in decompressing (although it is possible to do so if a feeding tube long enough to hold open the valve is used) and clogging of the valve (generally after 4–6 months). A recent report on the use of buttons in 50 children over a 20-month period describes a generally positive experience and makes recommendations for the use of this device.[90]

### Respiratory Support During Feedings

Monitoring heart rate, respiratory rate, and oxygenation status (either by pulse oximetry or transcutaneous oxygen monitor) is standard practice during initial feeding attempts for the BPD infant. These parameters, as well as the infant's clinical reaction to the process, can yield valuable information about the success of the feeding or the need to change a specific technique. The nasal cannula taped under the nares should be implemented for any infant requiring oxygen delivery during feeding.

The use of oxygen to supplement growth should also be considered. It has recently been reported that if infants are weaned too early from supplemental oxygen at home, their growth slows substantially.[91] We have seen infants who were able to maintain oxygen saturations above 92 percent but, when weaned to room air, failed to gain weight during the next seven to ten days. These infants began to gain weight again when low-flow oxygen via a nasal cannula was reinstituted. Other respiratory care that can improve feeding behavior includes suctioning (particularly nares) prior to feeding and optimizing respiratory capacity with the use of bronchodilators (Chapter 4). Both interventions should be carried out 20–30 minutes prior to feeding to allow a rest period and time for the infant to disassociate the negative effects of the interventions from the feeding experience.

## Growth Potential for Infants with BPD

Several follow-up studies have reported the growth patterns of infants recovering from BPD. One found that at two years of age, the average weight of survivors of BPD whose birthweight had been less than 1,500 gm was in the third to tenth percentile, height ranged from the tenth to twenty-fifth percentile, and head circumference was close to the fiftieth percentile.[92] Another study found a similar pattern of growth delay, with 37 percent of the children at two years of age below the tenth percentile for weight and 25 percent below the tenth percentile for height.[93]

Recent research has attempted to determine the causes of the growth failure. Half of a study population of infants recovering from BPD exhibited growth failure at six months corrected age; the other half did not. The respiratory status of the infants with growth failure was generally more severe, although the work of breathing as measured by pulmonary function testing did not completely explain their elevated oxygen consumption. All infants studied received adequate caloric intake, and fecal losses of nutrients were not excessive in either group.[45,53] Infants with more severe BPD do seem to exhibit a high rate of growth failure that is not completely explained by the increased work of breathing; other metabolic factors such as protein-calorie malnutrition may therefore be important.

## Conclusion

Providing appropriate nutrition is a complex aspect of the care of infants with BPD throughout their course of illness. Each stage represents different challenges—from managing parenteral nutrition during the acute phase for the infant on assisted ventilation, to introducing and promoting tolerance of enteral nutrients during the intermediate stage, to establishing oral feeding for the infant during the chronic stage of the illness. Close monitoring of growth parameters is essential because there are many variations in growth patterns among infants with BPD, and it may be necessary to tailor each infant's nutritional care plan slightly differently to achieve optimal growth. Neonatal nurses can contribute greatly not only to individual patient management but also by exploring the many questions that remain about providing nutritional care to the infant with BPD.

## Acknowledgments

The authors wish to thank Arthur D'Harlingue, MD and Linda Lefrak-Okikawa RN, MS for their helpful suggestions during preparation of this manuscript and Ms. Loretta Ross for secretarial assistance.

## References

1. Oh W: Nutritional management of infants with bronchopulmonary dysplasia, *in* Bronchopulmonary Dysplasia and Related Chronic Respiratory Disorders, Ninetieth Ross Conference of Pediatric Research, Ross Laboratories, 1986, Columbus, Ohio pp. 96–105.
2. Tooley W: Epidemiology of bronchopulmonary dysplasia, Journal of Pediatrics 95, 1979, pp. 851–855.
3. Spitzer A, Fox W, and Papadopoulos M: Maximum diuresis—a factor in predicting recovery from respiratory distress syndrome and the development of bronchopulmonary dysplasia, Journal of Pediatrics 98(3), March 1981, pp. 476–479.
4. Northway W, Rosan R, and Porter D: Pulmonary disease following respirator therapy of hyaline membrane disease: Bronchopulmonary dysplasia, New England Journal of Medicine 276, 1967, pp. 357–368.
5. Yeh T, et al.: Oxygen consumption and insensible water loss in premature infants in single- versus double-walled incubators, Journal of Pediatrics 97(6), 1980, pp. 967–971.

6. Baumgart S, Fox W, and Polin R: Physiologic implications of two different heat shields for infants under radiant warmers, Journal of Pediatrics 100, 1982, pp. 787–790.
7. Harpin V, and Rutter N: Humidification of incubator, Archives of Disease in Childhood 60, 1985, pp. 219–224.
8. Slotkin S, Bryon M, and Anderson G: Intravenous nitrogen and energy intakes required to duplicate in utero nitrogen accretion in prematurely born human infants, Journal of Pediatrics 99, 1981, pp. 115–120.
9. Kerner J, ed.: Manual of Pediatric Parenteral Nutrition, New York, 1983, Wiley.
10. Friedman A, et al.: Rapid onset of essential fatty acid deficiency in the newborn, Pediatrics 58, 1976, pp. 640–649.
11. Spear M, et al.: The effect of fifteen hour fat infusions of varying dosage on bilirubin binding to albumin, Journal of Parenteral and Enteral Nutrition 9, 1985, pp. 114–147.
12. Shennan A, et al.: The effect of intralipid on the elimination of serum bilirubin in the newborn infant, Journal of Pediatrics 88, 1976, pp. 285–288.
13. Bians Y, et al.: Fat emulsion tolerance in very low birth weight neonates: Effect on diffusion of oxygen in the lungs and on blood pH, Pediatrics 78(1), July 1986, pp. 79–84.
14. Kao L, Cheng M, and Warburton D: Triglycerides, free fatty acids/albumin molar ratio, and cholesterol levels in serum of neonates receiving long-term lipid infusions: Controlled trial of continuous and intermittent regimens, Journal of Pediatrics 104, March 1984, pp. 429–434.
15. Schreiner R, et al.: An evaluation of methods to monitor infants receiving intravenous lipids, Journal of Pediatrics 94, 1977, pp. 197–200.
16. D'Harlingue A, et al.: Limited value of nephelometry in monitoring the administration of intravenous fat in neonates, Journal of Parenteral and Enteral Nutrition 7, 1983, pp. 55–58.
17. Pieldes R, and Pyati S: Hypoglycemia and hyperglycemia in tiny infants, Clinics in Perinatology 13(2), June 1986, pp. 351–375.
18. Vaucher Y, Watson P, and Morrow G: Continuous insulin infusion in hyperglycemic, very low birth weight infants, Journal of Pediatric Gastroenterology and Nutrition 1(2), 1982, pp. 211–217.
19. Ostertag SG, et al.: Insulin pump therapy in very low birth weight infants, Pediatrics 78, 1986, pp. 625–630.
20. Pollak A, et al.: Glucose disposal in low-birth-weight infants during steady state hyperglycemia: Effects of exogenous insulin administration, Pediatrics 61, 1978, pp. 546–549.
21. Shannon L: Insulin usage in the neonate, Neonatal Network 6(5), April 1988, pp. 31–39.
22. Goldman S, and Hirata T: Attenuated response to insulin in very low birth weight infants, Pediatric Research 14, 1980, pp. 50–53.
23. Wilson D, Rogers R, and Hoffman R: Nutrition and chronic lung disease, American Review of Respiratory Disease 132, 1985, pp. 1347–1365.
24. Askanazi J, et al.: Respiratory changes induced by the large glucose loads of total parenteral nutrition, Journal of the American Medical Association 243, 1980, pp. 1444–1447.
25. Askanazi J, et al.: Respiratory distress secondary to a high carbohydrate load: A case report, Surgery 87, 1980, pp. 596–598.

26. Askanazi J, et al.: Nutrition for the patient with respiratory failure: Glucose versus fat, Anesthesiology 54, 1981, pp. 373–377.
27. Farrell M, and Balisteri W: Parenteral nutrition and hepatobiliary dysfunction, Clinics in Perinatology 13(1), March 1986, pp. 197–212.
28. Ekrenkranz RA, et al.: Amelioration of bronchopulmonary dysplasia after vitamin E administration: A preliminary report, New England Journal of Medicine 299, 1978, pp. 564–569.
29. Saldanha R, Cepeda E, and Poland R: The effect of vitamin E prophylaxis on the incidence and severity of bronchopulmonary dysplasia, Journal of Pediatrics 101, 1982, pp. 89–93.
30. Greene H, et al.: Evaluation of a pediatric multiple vitamin preparation for total parenteral nutrition, II: Blood level of vitamins A, D, and E, Pediatrics 77(4), April 1986, pp. 539–547.
31. Shenai J, Chytil F, and Stahlman M: Vitamin A status of neonates with bronchopulmonary dysplasia, Pediatric Research 19(2), 1985, pp. 185–189.
32. Shenai J, Chytil F, and Stahlman M: Liver vitamin A reserves of very low birth weight neonates, Pediatric Research 19(2), 1985, pp. 892–893.
33. Brandt R, et al.: Serum vitamin A in premature and term neonates, Journal of Pediatrics 92, 1978, pp. 101–104.
34. Shenai J, et al.: Plasma vitamin A and retinal binding protein in premature and term neonates, Journal of Pediatrics 99, 1981, pp. 302–305.
35. Hustead V, et al.: Relationship of vitamin A (retinol) status to lung disease in the preterm infant, Journal of Pediatrics 105(4), October 1984, pp. 610–615.
36. Shenai J, et al.: Clinical trial of vitamin A supplementation in infants susceptible to bronchopulmonary dysplasia, Journal of Pediatrics 111(2), August 1987, pp. 269–277.
37. Hartline J, and Zachman R: Vitamin A delivery in total parenteral nutrition solution, Pediatrics 58, 1976, pp. 448–451.
38. Shenai J, Stahlman M, and Chytil F: Vitamin A delivery from parenteral alimentation solution, Journal of Pediatrics 99, 1981, pp. 661–663.
39. Greene H, Phillip B, and Franck L: Persistently low blood retinol levels during and after parenteral feedings of very low birth weight infants: Examination of losses into intravenous administration sets and a method of prevention by addition to a lipid emulsion, Pediatrics 79(6), June 1987, pp. 894–900.
40. Steichen J, Gratton T, and Tsang R: Osteopenia of prematurity: The cause and possible treatment, Journal of Pediatrics 96, 1980, pp. 528–534.
41. Durand M, et al.: Prospective evaluation of percutaneous central venous silastic catheters in newborn infants with birth weights of 510–3,920 grams, Pediatrics 78(2), August 1986, pp. 245–250.
42. Chathas MK: Percutaneous central venous catheters in neonates, Journal of Obstetric, Gynecologic, and Neonatal Nursing 15(4), July/August 1986, pp. 324–332.
43. Lefrak L, et al.: Catheter life, infection rate and complication associated with the use of percutaneously inserted silastic venous catheters in neonates, Clinical Research 32, 1984, p. 126A.

44. Weinstein M, and Oh W: Oxygen consumption in infants with bronchopulmonary dysplasia, Journal of Pediatrics 99, 1981, pp. 958–961.

45. Kurzner S, et al.: Growth failure in bronchopulmonary dysplasia: Elevated metabolic rates and pulmonary mechanics, Journal of Pediatrics 112(1), January 1988, pp. 73–80.

46. Schulman R, et al.: Protein deficiency in premature infants receiving parenteral nutrition, American Journal of Clinical Nutrition 44, 1986, pp. 610–613.

47. Morris F, et al.: Ontogenic development of gastrointestinal motility IV: Duodenal contractions in preterm infants, Pediatrics 78(6), December 1986, pp. 1106–1113.

48. Heldt G: The effect of gavage feeding on the mechanics of the lung, chest wall, and diaphragm of preterm infants, Pediatric Research 24 (1), 1988, pp. 55–58.

49. Greer F, et al.: Changes in fat concentration of human milk during delivery by intermittent bolus and continuous mechanical pump infusion, Journal of Pediatrics 105(5), November 1984, pp. 745–749.

50. Bhatin J, and Fomon S: Formulas for premature infants: Fate of calcium and phosphorous, Pediatrics 72(1), July 1983, pp. 37–40.

51. Goodwin S, Graves S, and Haberkern C: Aspiration in intubated infants, Pediatrics 75(1), January 1985, pp. 85–88.

52. Pereira G, and Hemons J: Controlled study of transpyloric and intermittent gavage feeding in the small preterm infant, Pediatrics 67(1), January 1981, pp. 68–72.

53. Kurzner S, et al.: Growth failure in infants with bronchopulmonary dysplasia: Nutrition and elevated resting metabolic expenditure, Pediatrics 81(3), March 1988, pp. 379–384.

54. Callenbach J, et al.: Etiological factors in rickets of very low birth weight infants, Journal of Pediatrics 98, 1981, pp. 800–805.

55. Chudley A, et al.: Nutritional rickets in two very low birth weight infants with chronic lung disease, Archives of Disease in Childhood 55, 1980, pp. 687–690.

56. Hrabovsky E, and Mullett M: Gastroesophageal reflux and the premature infant, Journal of Pediatric Surgery 21(7), July 1986, pp. 583–587.

57. Euler A, et al.: Recurrent pulmonary disease in children: A complication of gastroesophageal reflux, Pediatrics 63(1), January 1979, pp. 47–51.

58. Herbst J: Gastroesophageal reflux, Journal of Pediatrics 98(6), 1981, pp. 859–870.

59. Herbst J, Book L, and Bray P: Gastroesophageal reflux in the "near miss" sudden infant death syndrome, Journal of Pediatrics 92(1), January 1978, pp. 73–75.

60. Herbst J, Minton S, and Book L: Gastroesophageal reflux causing respiratory distress and apnea in newborn infants, Journal of Pediatrics 95(5), November 1979, pp. 763–768.

61. Johnson D: Current thinking on the role of surgery in gastroesophageal reflux, Pediatric Clinics of North America 32(5), October 1985, pp. 1165–1179.

62. Orenstein S, Whitington P, and Orenstein D: The infant seat as treatment for gastroesophageal reflux, New England Journal of Medicine 309(13), September 29, 1983, pp. 760–763.

63. Orenstein S, and Whitington P: Positioning for prevention of infant gastroesophageal reflux, Journal of Pediatrics 103(4), October 1983, pp. 534–537.

64. Orenstein S, Magill H, and Brooks P: Thickening of infant feedings for therapy of gastroesophageal reflux, Journal of Pediatrics 110(2), February 1987, pp. 181–186.
65. Bailey D, et al.: Lack of efficacy of thickened feedings as treatment for gastroesophageal reflux, Journal of Pediatrics 110(2), February 1987, pp. 187–189.
66. Ulshen M: Treatment of gastroesophageal reflux: Is nothing sacred? (commentary), Journal of Pediatrics 110(2), February 1987, pp. 254–255.
67. Sasso S: Metaclopromide and chalasia, The American Journal of Maternal-Child Nursing 8, September/October 1983, p. 361.
68. Machida H, et al.: Metoclopromide in gastroesophageal reflux of infancy, Journal of Pediatrics 112(3), March 1988, pp. 483–487.
69. Galley S, et al.: Postoperative small bowel obstruction in infants and children: A problem following Nissen fundoplication, Journal of Pediatric Surgery 21(5), May 1986, pp. 407–409.
70. Gryboski J, and Walker A, eds.: Suck and swallow, (chapter 1) *in* Gastrointestinal Problems in the Infant, Philadelphia, 1975, W.B. Saunders, pp. 17–47.
71. Guilleminault C, and Coons S: Apnea and bradycardia during feedings in infants weighing <2000 gm, Journal of Pediatrics 104 (6), pp. 932–935.
72. Garg M, et al.: Clinically unsuspected hypoxia during sleep and feeding in infants with bronchopulmonary dysplasia, Pediatrics 81 (5), May 1988, pp. 635–642.
73. Feldman S, Deal C, and Urquhart W: Disturbance of swallowing after tracheostomy, Lancet 1, 1966, pp. 954–955.
74. Braun M, and Palmer M: A pilot study of oral-motor dysfunction in "at risk" infants, Physical and Occupational Therapy in Pediatrics 5(4), Winter 1985/1986, pp. 13–25.
75. Blackman J, and Nelson C: Reinstituting oral feedings in children fed by gastrostomy tube, Clinical Pediatrics 24(8), August 1985, pp. 434–438.
76. Geertsma M, et al.: Feeding resistance after parenteral hyperalimentation, American Journal of Diseases of Children 139, March 1985, pp. 255–256.
77. Zisserman L: Feeding problems: Weaning an infant from a transpyloric tube, Pediatric Nursing 12(1), January/February 1988, pp. 33–37.
78. Ardran G, and Kemp F: Some important factors in the assessment of oropharyngeal function, Developmental Medicine and Child Neurology 12, 1970, pp. 158–166.
79. Hambridge K: Low levels of zinc in hair, anorexia, poor growth and hypogeusia in children, Pediatric Research 6, 1972, pp. 868–874.
80. Meier P, and Anderson G: Responses of small preterm infants to bottle- and breastfeeding, The American Journal of Maternal-Child Nursing 12, 1987, pp. 97–105.
81. Meier P: Bottle-and breastfeeding: Effects on transcutaneous oxygen pressure and temperature in preterm infants, Nursing Research 37 (1), 1988, pp. 36–41.
82. Marmet C, and Shell E: Training neonates to suck correctly, The American Journal of Maternal-Child Nursing 9, November/December 1984, pp. 401–407.
83. Schulze K, et al.: Energy expenditure, energy balance, and composition of weight gain in low birth weight infants fed diets of different protein and energy content, Journal of Pediatrics 110(5), May 1987, pp. 753–759.
84. Cavell B: Effect of feeding an infant formula with high energy density on gastric emptying in infants with congenital heart disease, Acta Paediatrica Scandinavica 70, 1981, pp. 513–516.

85. Cavell B: Gastric emptying in infants with congenital heart disease, Acta Paediatrica Scandinavica 70, 1981, pp. 517–520.

86. Ohio Neonatal Nutritionists: Bronchopulmonary dysplasia, *in* Nutritional Care for High Risk Newborns, Philadelphia, 1985, George F. Stickley, pp. 170–179.

87. Nutrient Values of Gerber Baby Foods 1987, Professional Communications Department, Gerber Products Company, Fremont, Michigan.

88. Fisher S, Painter M, and Milmoe G: Swallowing disorder in infancy, Pediatric Clinics of North America 28(4), 1981, pp. 845–853.

89. Huth M, and O'Brien M: The gastrostomy feeding button™, Pediatric Nursing 13(4), August 1987, pp. 241–245.

90. Gauderer M, et al.: Feeding gastrostomy button: Experience and recommendations, Journal of Pediatric Surgery 23(1), January 1988, pp. 24–28.

91. Groothius J, and Rosenberg A: Home oxygen promotes weight gain in infants with bronchopulmonary dysplasia, Pediatrics 74, 1984, pp. 217–220.

92. Markestad T, and Fitzhardinge P: Growth and development in children recovering from bronchopulmonary dysplasia, Journal of Pediatrics 98(4), April 1981, pp. 597–602.

93. Yu V, et al.: Growth and development of very low birth weight infants recovering from bronchopulmonary dysplasia, Archives of Disease in Childhood 58, 1983, pp. 791–794.

CHAPTER 6

# Behavioral Issues for Infants with BPD

*Kathleen A. VandenBerg, MA*
*Children's Hospital*
*Oakland, California*

*Linda S. Franck, RN, MS*
*Children's Hospital*
*Oakland, California*

There are many complex associations between the behavior manifested by an infant with bronchopulmonary dysplasia (BPD) and physiologic compromise. This chapter describes some of the typical behaviors of the infant with BPD and suggests specific strategies for environmental, behavioral, and pharmacologic intervention. These strategies are designed to help reduce the stressful stimuli inherent in the intensive care nursery environment in order to enhance recovery and ensure improved developmental outcome.

### The Problem

Severe BPD almost invariably means a prolonged and complicated hospital course.[1] The impact of prolonged illness requiring restriction of movement, exposure to high levels of inappropriate patterns of sensory input, and loss of a consistent primary caregiver can mean deleterious adaptation patterns that can lead to distortions in functioning.[2-4] Developmental morbidity studies have shown a more encouraging outcome for full-term and large premature infants who require mechanical ventilation, but studies of infants weighing less than 1,500 gm who require assisted ventilation indicate a 45 percent incidence of handicaps.[5–9] The sicker the infant, the higher the risk of poor developmental outcome. Infants who develop chronic lung disease have a prolonged recovery and frequently exhibit pulmonary symptoms up to eight years of age.[7,10]

Impediments to planning and implementing developmentally appropriate care for these infants fall into three main areas: (1) lack of obvious cues from the infant to warn of impending agitation leading to physiologic compromise, (2) inability to organize bedside care around the unpredictability of the infant's state, and (3) lack of interventions to effectively soothe these infants.

The instability of the infant's behavioral control is a major factor contributing to the stress of caring for the BPD infant. The infant may be in deep sleep and within seconds become agitated and hypoxic for no readily apparent reason. The infant's nurse often has little warning prior to emesis or need for suctioning. The frequently sudden buildup of irritability or of secretions makes it extremely difficult to plan or organize care for such an unpredictable patient. To compound the problem, the nurse may be caring for one or two other infants who may be equally unpredictable, with episodes that could result in severe compromise for any of these patients.

Many times the interventions used to try to soothe the agitated infant before he aspirates or has a bronchospasm will be unsuccessful. These infants do not usually respond to typical soothing techniques such as rocking, patting, holding, or talking. Interventions that have proven successful for one nurse at one time may not work for nurses on other shifts caring for the same infant. It is understandable that these infants soon gain quite a reputation among the nursing staff and seem to sense the fear and tension of the nurse who is caring for them for the first time. Care of the infant with BPD can be an unrewarding experience for even the most dedicated NICU nurse because neither the infant's nor the caregiver's needs are met.

The frustrations of caring for the BPD infant can spill over and affect the working relationships among the members of the health care team. Differences in perception of the problem, expectations, goals, and coping strategies among members of the health care team increase the likelihood of conflict. Breakdowns in communication are not uncommon and must be addressed if the team's efforts are to be effective.

A major source of concern and potential conflict is the problem of infant agitation and the use of sedatives for its management. In a national study of intensive care nurseries, 95 percent of the respondents reported that management of agitation was a problem in their unit.[11] Variations in approach to the problem, lack of knowledge, and inconsistent or inappropriate use of pharmacologic agents compound the problem. Effective medical and nursing care for these infants is predicated on the realization that the infant with BPD is one of the most complex and challenging patients seen in the NICU today.

To parents, the diagnosis of BPD can mean increasing the stress in their lives by a lengthened hospitalization for the child they have yet to bring home. These parents are burdened with added health care expenses, increased family anxiety, and prolonged uncertainty about the ultimate survival and developmental outcome of their infant. Parents often report feelings of helplessness and inadequacy as they attempt to establish some form of human interaction with their very fragile infant. Behavior typical of the BPD infant includes squirming or arching when held and crying or turning away when parents attempt to make face-to-face contact. The infant's behavior often develops into a pattern of unrewarding feedback to the parent whose limits of frustration may have already been exceeded.

The developmental outcome of the premature infant has been shown to be determined more by the parent-infant relationship and the social milieu than by any other factors. This first relationship serves as the basis for all later learning and assists the infant as he negotiates his world in the first three to five years of life. Given the importance of a healthy parent-infant relationship to good developmental outcome, helping the parent acquire the necessary competence in the vital role of primary caretaker is an essential component of nursing care.

## Improved Outcome with Intervention

We are on the brink of learning through research about the efficacy of developmental interventions in the NICU. In one study conducted by Als and associates, 16 infants at risk for BPD were studied to determine if carefully individualized behavioral recommendations to reduce stress and organize the infant's self-regulatory abilities were beneficial. The ventilator dependent infants were less than 28 weeks gestational age and weighed less than 1,250 gm at birth. The control and intervention groups showed no significant differences on any of the medical (oxygen requirements during first 48 hours and the first ten days, patent ductus arteriosus, and intraventricular hemorrhage) or demographic variables (maternal age, parity, socioeconomic status, and ethnicity).[12]

The control group received routine care in the NICU with primary nurses as caregivers. The experimental group received specifically scheduled assessments of infant stress levels during caregiving every tenth day. In the experimental group, primary care nurses were given systematic feedback suggestions in how to read the infant's subtle cues. They were also shown how to institute the best modes of supporting the infant's behavioral organization, which meant organizing all caregiving routines to coincide with each infant's awake states.[12]

There were significant differences between the experimental and control groups. The experimental group was on the ventilator an average of 35 days less than the control group, received supplemental oxygen an average of 29 days less than the control group, and graduated to complete bottle/breast-feeding an average of 45 days sooner than the control group. The experimental infants also showed significant improvement over the controls in developmental functioning at one, three, six, and nine months corrected age. The researchers attribute these results to the management of stress in these BPD infants and the *timing* of caregiving routines to support infant behavioral organization.[12]

In a replication of this study by Als and her colleagues with 18 control and 20 experimental infants, experimental infants achieved similar gains as those in the previous study, including: significantly shorter ventilator courses, fewer days on support oxygen, earlier establishment of breast/bottle feeds, improved average daily weight gain, lower incidence of intraventricular hemorrhage, younger age at discharge and shorter hospital stay. The experimental group also experienced reduced severity of BPD. Als estimated that approximately $90,000 was saved in hospital costs for EACH experimental infant in this second study.[13]

In order to optimize the experience of infants with BPD in the NICU and provide the necessary support to reduce stress and improve interactions, an understanding of their behavior is essential. A model of preterm development that describes the emerging early behavioral organization of the preterm infant has been developed by Als and colleagues.[14–17] The synactive theory of development is based on the assumption that the infant's primary route of communicating his thresholds of stress or his functional stability is through his behavior.

For the infant with BPD (whether premature or full-term), this model provides a systematic catalogue of behavior that can help caregivers describe and understand the infant's individual signals of stress or stability. Describing these individual signs allows the neonatal nurse to begin to plan appropriate intervention strategies, modify the environment, or alter handling techniques in order to reinstitute a balanced integrated state and prevent excessive agitation in infants with BPD.[13–18]

In using this model to evaluate the level of function of the preterm infant Als postulates that we first need to determine the level of development and integrity of each system—including the autonomic system, the motor system, the state system, and the attention and self-regulatory systems.[15,16] The autonomic system can be seen in the pattern of respiration (pauses, tachypnea), color changes (red, pale, dusky, mottled), and various visceral signs (emesis, seizures, twitching). The motor system is seen by observing the infant's posture (hyperflexed, flaccid, extended), specific movement patterns (of extremities, trunk, head, face), and level of activity. The state system is seen in the available range of the states of consciousness (from sleep, arousal, awake and alert to crying). The states may be poorly defined at first with, for example, jerky body twitches and fussing accompanying sleep and awake states. The attention system is seen in the infant's ability to orient and focus on sensory stimuli in the outside milieu such as face, sounds, or objects. The self-regulatory system is seen in the behaviors the infant uses to maintain the integrity and balance of the other systems. Some infants can tuck their limbs in close to their body in an effort to gain control if stressed; others seem to relax if they can brace a foot against the side of the crib.

Questions for the caregiver to consider include the following: At what level of environmental demand does the infant lose control? At what level can he cope adequately, and which behaviors indicate the first signs of loss of control? At what point is intervention needed? Which strategies are useful to bring about a relaxed integrated balance between the subsystems and reduce stress, thus freeing up calories for growth and neurodevelopment?

## Behavioral Manifestations of Stress

Many of the complex associations between the infant's behavior and manifestations of physiologic compromise have not been well described. Several of the behavioral issues emerge repeatedly as one considers the daily experience of the infant with BPD. The increased work of breathing, the emotional and social deprivation from being severely ill for a long time, and confinement to a hospital bed for months in an environment with an inappropriate pattern of stimuli contribute to the behavioral manifestations of stress.[2] Such behaviors, which are described in the following sections, interfere with the normal process of development and may severely impair the infant's ability to interact.

### Excessive Energy Expenditures

At many times during the course of BPD, the amount of energy available to the infant for interaction with his environment will be limited. During the acute phase of the disease, caloric intake is limited, and the physiologic expenditures are great. Maintenance of heart rate, blood pressure, and respiration requires significant energy. If the infant at any time is not adequately oxygenated, the energy will be provided by anaerobic metabolism that puts the infant at an overall deficit.

Studies have shown that crying, supine positioning, excessive handling, jarring loud noises, poorly timed social interactions, and poorly organized sleep states can affect the oxygenation of the preterm infant with respiratory disease.[4,19–22] Even during the convalescent phase of BPD, energy requirements of tissue growth and repair are increased. Oxygen consumption in infants with BPD has been reported in one study to be 25 percent greater than infants of the same age without BPD.[23] Nurses describe these infants as having "no reserves" to meet the demands of the environment.

With such a precarious balance between metabolic requirements and energy intake, any environmental stressor, no matter how innocuous, can precipitate a setback in the infant's medical condition. A sick infant's level of responsiveness is often expressed first by autonomic signs rather than on an interactive level.[4] Even turning the infant or changing a diaper can precipitate a hypoxic episode in the BPD infant who has little or no energy reserves. As a result, more oxygen must then be delivered at a higher rate and/or pressure to prevent further tissue hypoxia and acidosis.

Sometimes the effects are cumulative: The infant may appear to tolerate a procedure such as a spinal tap but then become apneic and cyanotic when a blood gas is drawn ten minutes later. The cumulative effect of such experiences can result in longer recovery from each episode, leaving the infant severely depleted of energy unless oxygen or ventilatory support is increased. The infant may appear to tolerate procedures performed over a period of days and then appear to suddenly "crash." By systematically decreasing external stressors, the health care team can reduce the amount of behavioral energy expended by the infant thus releasing energy for growth and tissue repair.[23]

## Overreactivity

When observing the BPD infant's reactions to stimuli, one typically sees a consistently low threshold for stress. As the infant reacts to a stimulus, his reaction often results in an avalanche of activity, becoming at times uncontrolled. The stress can be seen as physiological instability (increased or decreased heart rate or respiratory rate) or motor disorganization (flailing, tremors, arching) or changes in state control (abruptly becoming irritable or sleepy). The infant, even after a short period of handling, may be flaccid, exhausted, and physiologically compromised as a result of sensory overload.[4,14–18]

### Poor Self-Regulation

The infant with BPD characteristically has a paucity of physiological, postural, or state system strategies to maintain himself. He may be so stressed that he can no longer make any effort to react to stimulation. As he slowly begins to recover from his BPD, efforts to regulate himself may be seen, although they frequently are unsuccessful. For example, an infant who is positioned supine after a stressful procedure such as suctioning struggles to turn and pull his limbs into a flexed posture. He will try to flex and eventually become exhausted, too weak to try. At this point, he is very vulnerable to the caregiver's handling. The infant who is further along in recovery and has developed self-regulatory skills may be able to briefly achieve but not successfully maintain himself in a preferred posture. The infant with good self-control will not only successfully maintain a preferred posture, but may have developed a repertoire of several postures he can use to calm or relax himself.[15,18]

### Recycling

This reaction is seen in the infant's motor system as he reacts to a stimulus. The reaction can be one of ongoing repetition of motor behaviors such as flailing or arching. This can set up an escalating pattern, which again the infant cannot control or stop. The integrity of the physiological system is eventually affected, and this may result in a hypoxic event or apnea.[16]

### Defensive Behaviors

Several patterns of avoidance or defensiveness are observable in the infant with BPD and can manifest themselves through each subsystem. Defensive behaviors can include gagging, hiccoughs, grimacing, spitting up, arching, fingersplay, airplaning, arm/leg extensions, sitting on air, sneezing, yawning, sighing, coughing, averting, and frowning.[16]

Eventually, approach or orienting behavior develops, and the infant's task is to smoothly integrate and regulate both approach and avoidance behaviors.[16] For the BPD infant, the avoidance maneuvers may be preponderant as he attempts to defend himself against inappropriately timed or inappropriately intense or complex stimuli. This behavior should be viewed as a strength as the infant struggles to control physiological components (particularly respirations) along with posture, movement, and state. For example, as the infant begins to open his eyes, the caregiver (understandably excited after many days or weeks of viewing a sleepy or irritable infant) presents his or her face in close range to encourage social interchange. This is often met with immediate eye shutting or turning away; or if the infant is acutely stressed, respirations may fluctuate dramatically, and he will become pale or even dusky.

Many times the infant can tolerate only a very low level of stimulation presented *one stimulus at a time*. When these defensive behaviors are respected, the skilled caregiver can eventually elicit effective face-to-face interaction. If these defensive behaviors are not well understood by the caregiver, these otherwise temporary actions can become entrenched patterns and interfere with the acquisition of competent social and interactive skills at a later stage.

### Frantic Activity

BPD infants can express stress as frantic, diffuse activity. They often react as if in a panicked state as they abruptly become irritable. They seem to have a sense of fear that may come from being "air hungry" or unsure about their breathing capacity. This stress is observable and can be managed by the individualized environmental strategies discussed later. The goal is to recognize this behavior as soon as possible and intervene to prevent its escalation. Frequent and prolonged frantic activity evolves into a condition of agitation.

### Agitation

Agitation is considered a problem in many NICU patients today. In a survey by Franck,[11] neonatal nurses described agitation as consisting of crying (or cry face), increased activity, and irritability often accompanied by decreased oxygenation, duskiness, increased respiratory effort, and feeding intolerance. Infants with BPD were identified as being more at risk for agitation than infants with other diagnoses. The agitation was described as occurring frequently, disrupting feeding and sleep, and often compromising respiration. In 79 percent of the NICUs surveyed, sedatives were used to manage the agitation of the infant with chronic lung disease.

Although pain and distress due to unpleasant environmental stimuli can be components of the agitated condition, management of pain or manipulation of environmental factors alone may not resolve the agitated behavior. Agitation is the result of both internal and external factors affecting the infant who has an inherent or acquired hypersensitivity to stimuli. Behaviorally, agitation is manifest as irritability, increased gross motor activity, and restlessness.

Agitation severe enough to cause physiologic compromise is particularly of concern in the infant with BPD who has many serious physiologic stressors with which to contend. The relationship of hypoxia, acidosis, pain, increased respiratory secretions, bronchospasm, gastroesophageal reflux, and pharmacologic therapy to the agitated state of the infant must be considered. Bronchospasm, for example, is a complex phenomenon involving increased airway resistance and/or airway obstruction and hypoxemia. It is not known whether agitated behavior precipitates bronchospasm or bronchospasm causes the agitated behavior, but the two factors appear to be associated.[24] If the infant experiences frequent agitation that disrupts behavioral state, feeding, or effective oxygenation, the medical course may be even more prolonged and complex.

### Disruptive Feeding Behaviors

The physical skills required to ingest food begin to develop *in utero* and continue to advance through the first three years of life.[25] This development is the result of maturation of the central nervous system as well as a function of the child's interaction with his caregiver and environment. The early feeding environment can have a strong influence on the development of abnormal patterns.[26] Infants in home environments with consistent primary caregivers learn to eat through a series of repeated, pleasurable experiences. As a warm substance is introduced into the mouth, a loving caregiver holds the baby close, talks to and smiles at him, and gradually relieves the hunger pangs in the stomach.

Part of this process is learning to perceive and respond to the tactile stimulus from the food. Babies learn to tolerate feeding utensils and various food textures, then to initiate oral play with their own hands, bringing objects to the mouth repeatedly. Sucking in a rhythmic pattern of two sucks per breath becomes easily established, and coordination of the suck-suck-swallow-breathe pattern is effortless for a healthy full-term infant who has well-developed jaw and tongue movements.[25]

Prematurity interferes with the neurological and physical integrity of the moving parts needed to coordinate feeding and breathing. The premature infant is deprived of the full 40 weeks of *in utero* practice of sucking and swallowing. The physiologic flexion provided by compression of the amniotic sac, which helps keep oral mechanisms aligned properly, is missed. Vestibular sensations provided by the mother, which effect muscle tone and tactile and proprioceptive input to the body, face, and mouth, are limited.[25]

The premature infant's oral structures do not function like those of the full-term neonate. The oral cavity in the premature infant is small, and the jaw is often retracted. The tongue does not completely fill the oral cavity (as in the full term), and with extra space, air comes in, interfering with the suck-swallow-breathe pattern. The tongue and jaw movements are less controlled. Excessive jaw depression may be a problem, or the infant may not initiate any jaw movement at all when offered the nipple to suck. Often the infant cannot "cup" the tongue to control flow of liquid to the rear of the mouth for swallowing.[25] The tongue of the premature infant may be pulled back with the tip elevated, making nipple insertion difficult.

For the premature infant with BPD, normal, positive early feeding experiences are usually absent in the NICU environment. Invasive procedures such as intubation, passage of nasogastric tubes, and taping tubes to the face are noxious oral experiences that contribute to the onset of oral defensive behaviors such as hypersensitivity to touch. Pain may be paired with oral stimuli (when, for example, a pacifier is routinely offered during invasive procedures) so much that the infant is conditioned to respond negatively to any oral stimuli. Further research is required to understand the relationship, if any, between classical conditioning involving oral stimuli and subsequent maladaptive feeding patterns. One might hypothesize that once the infant has learned that oral experience is painful, effectively intervening to normalize oral motor responses may be extremely difficult.

The behavioral problem of poorly regulated neurobehavioral function in BPD infants is perhaps most evident at the point in recovery when oral feeding is introduced. Either the infant is too sleepy to rouse or nipples the first swallow and becomes apneic (or tachypneic), seeming to drown in the small flow of formula. Sucking cannot be sustained. At times, these infants may look as if they are sucking and swallowing well, but they often are stressed and gag, choke, and leak liquid as they suck. Nippling even small amounts can lead to exhaustion and flaccidity, and again the infant cannot regulate his respirations along with coordinated suck and swallow. Compounding the problem is anxiety over adequate weight gain; staff may have to be rigid about feeding schedules at the risk of offering food at times not compatible with the infant's readiness.

## Objectives of Behavioral Care

The following five major goals of nursing care for the BPD infant form the basis for intervention:

1. Reducing hypoxic episodes and behavior that precipitates physiologic compromise
2. Reducing negative environmental stimuli
3. Helping parents understand the stressed infant's behavior and develop a relationship that yields rewarding interactions during and after hospitalization
4. Improving developmental outcome through individualized behavioral interventions that support the infant's ability to manage stress and pro-

mote developmental competence

5. Reducing the hospital stay through improvement in physiologic and behavioral health

## Assessing Behavior of BPD Infants

Investigators have found that neonates, even stressed neonates, give cues to caregivers as to their wellbeing or tensions.[12,27] Learning to recognize these behavioral signals is an essential first step in improving the developmental care of the BPD infant. These cues may indicate either disorganized (stress) or smooth functioning (stability) behavior in the infant and are expressed via the five subsystems described earlier. Lists of stress and stability signals based on Als's catalogue of approach and avoidance behaviors for each subsystem have been devised (see Tables 1 and 2).[15] Sensitivity to these signs of stress or stability will provide the caregiver with an understanding of each infant's threshold for stimulation as well as a means of identifying disorganized behaviors.[28]

Many signs of stress may be expressed physiologically at first, before other systems mature. Recognition of the emerging signs of *effort* to control self and the *cost* of making that effort is also important.[4,14,16,29] High and Gorski found that stress signs in NICU infants could occur at least five minutes *after* an intervention by a nurse and that chronically ill infants received less than three minutes observation time by nurses following interventions.[30] They concluded that nurses may be missing the chance to observe the causal relationship between the intervention and the infant's response.

One nurse in our NICU was astonished when it was pointed out that an increase in mild apneic spells was associated with the technique she used to turn the infant over because the apneic episodes occurred 4.75 minutes following the intervention. When she was shown how to rotate the baby slowly and gently with his limbs contained, mild apnea ceased. By remaining at the bedside longer, she was able to observe the effect of the intervention.

The first step in planning a behavioral intervention care plan is assessing the infant's responses to typical procedures and events in the NICU. Assessment of infant responses should include observation of the infant's physiological status, state, and activity level before, during, and after a typical NICU event. The NIDCAP (Neonatal Individualized Developmental Care and Assessment Program) is a formal certification program offered by Dr. Heideleise Als (see Appendix C). It provides training in assessing the developmental needs of high-risk infants and in structuring their care. Other informal assessment and planning strategies may also be effective if carried out thoroughly and regularly revised during an infant's hospital course. A systematic

**TABLE 1 ■ Signs of Stress in ICN Infants (Derived from: Assessment of Preterm Infant Behavior, Als, 1982)**

| AUTONOMIC SYSTEM | MOTOR SYSTEM | STATE SYSTEM (RANGE) | ATTENTION-INTERACTION SYSTEM | SELF-REGULATORY SYSTEM |
|---|---|---|---|---|
| ***Respiration:***<br>pauses, tachypnea, gasping<br>***Color Changes:***<br>paling around nostrils, peri-oral duskiness, mottled, cyanotic, gray, flushed, ruddy<br>***Visceral:***<br>hiccups, gagging, grunting, spitting up;<br>straining as if actually producing a bowel movement<br>***Motor:***<br>seizures<br>tremoring/startling<br>twitching<br>coughing<br>sneezing<br>yawning<br>sighing | ***Fluctuating Tone:***<br>Flaccidity of<br>• trunk<br>• extremities<br>• face<br>***Hypertonicity:***<br>• leg extensions<br>• salutes<br>• airplaning<br>• sitting on air<br>• arching<br>• finger splays<br>• tongue extensions<br>• fisting<br>***Hyperflexions:***<br>• trunk<br>• extremities<br>• fetal tuck<br>***Frantic, diffuse activity*** | ***Diffuse states:***<br>Sleep:<br>• twitches<br>• sounds<br>• jerky moves<br>• irregular respirations<br>• whimpers<br>• grimacing<br>• fussy in sleep<br>***Awake:***<br>• eye floating<br>• glassy eyed<br>• strained fussy<br>• staring<br>• gaze aversion<br>• panicked, worried or dull look<br>• weak cry<br>• irritability<br>• abrupt state changes | ***May demonstrate stress signals of other systems:***<br>• irregular respirations<br>• color changes<br>• visceral responses<br>• coughing, twitches,<br>• sneezing<br>• yawning<br>• sighing<br>• eye floating<br>• glassy eyed<br>• staring<br>• straining<br>• gaze aversion<br>• panicked, worried or dull look<br>• weak cry<br>• irritability<br>• abrupt state changes<br>• fluctuating tone<br>• frantic, diffuse activity<br>• becomes stressed with more than one mode of stimuli | ***May use the following to attempt to gain balance:***<br>• lowers state<br>• postural changes<br>• motoric strategies leg/foot bracing, hand clasping, foot clasping, finger folding, hand to mouth, sucking, grasping, hand holding, tucking<br>• good self-quieting & consolability<br>• rhythmic, robust crying<br>• clear sleep state<br>• focused alertness with: shiny-eyed and focused attention, animated expression, frowning, cheek softening, "ooh" face, cooing, smiling |
| **INTERVENTION STRATEGIES TO REDUCE STRESS** | | | | |
| Modify environment (light, noise, traffic)<br>Positioning<br>Minimal handling<br>Swaddling/covering | Positioning<br>Handling to contain limbs<br>Handling slow/gentle<br>Blanket rolls<br>Containment, nesting | Clustering care<br>Primary nursing to accurately read infant cues<br>Appropriate timing of activities and daily routines<br>Autonomic & Motoric subsystems must have reached stability | Modulate interactions to infant's tolerance level.<br>Provide supports necessary to bring out best alertness<br>Offer 1 mode of stimulation at a time<br>Use modulated voice, face, rattle, face and voice together<br>(Baby responds best to animate stimuli) | Provide support<br>• hold hand<br>• hold foot<br>Modify interactions<br>Modify environment<br>Swaddle<br>Organize daily routine to infant's best times |

**TABLE 2 ■ Signs of Stability (Derived from: Assessment of Preterm Infant Behavior, Als, 1982)**

| AUTONOMIC SYSTEM | MOTOR SYSTEM | STATE SYSTEM | ATTENTION SYSTEM | SELF-REGULATORY SYSTEM |
|---|---|---|---|---|
| Smooth, regular respirations<br>Pink, stable color<br>Stable viscera with no evidence of:<br>• seizures<br>• gagging<br>• emesis<br>• grunting<br>• tremors<br>• startles<br>• twitches<br>• coughing<br>• sneezing<br>• yawning<br>• sighing | Smooth, controlled posture<br>Smooth movements of extremities, head seen in:<br>• hand clasp<br>• leg/foot bracing<br>• foot clasp<br>• finger folding<br>• hand to mouth<br>• grasping<br>• sucking<br>• tucking<br>• hand holding<br>Good consistent tone throughout body | Clear, well-defined sleep states<br>Good self-quieting & consolability<br>Robust crying<br>Focused, clear alertness with animated expressions such as:<br>• frowning<br>• cheek softening<br>• "ooh" face<br>• cooing<br>• smiling | Responsivity to auditory and visual stimuli bright and of long duration<br>Actively seeks out auditory and shifts attention smoothly on his own from one stimulus to another<br>Face demonstrates bright-eyed purposeful interest varying between arousal and relaxation | Infant has sophisticated, well differentiated repertoire of successful strategies to maintain each system: autonomic, motor, state, and attention, such as:<br>*autonomic:* sucking, grasping<br>*motor:* tucking, foot bracing<br>*state:* visual locking, sucking<br>*attention:* hand to mouth, hand holding |

**INTERVENTIONS**

Interventions not necessary to reduce stress; but to enhance and facilitate normal development.

**TABLE 3 ▪ Minimal Handling Protocol**

***Protect from Light***
- Shade infant's eyes (with blanket "tent" or cutout box)
- Cover incubator with blankets
- Cover crib with blankets

***Protect from Noise***
- Give shift report away from the bedside
- Ensure that phones do not ring in nursery rooms
- Pad all trash receptacles
- Close incubator doors gently
- Set intercom volume levels as low as possible
- Close doors softly
- Remove sources of loud, jarring noise
- Avoid tearing paper near infant

***Protect from Overstimulation***
- Cluster nursing care activities
- Allow 2–3 hour periods of undisturbed rest
- No routine postural drainage (PRN only)
- No routine suctioning (PRN only)
- Contain limbs during suctioning (swaddle or have another person help)

*Note:* Allow for recovery after each intervention

***Provide Boundaries***
- Position prone or side lying
- Cover/wrap/swaddle
- Use blanket rolls to tuck around sides/back/feet even at head
- Provide objects for suck, grasp

observation would enable the observer to answer the following questions:

1. What are the baseline parameters of vital signs, state ranges, and activity level for this infant before handling begins?
2. What changes were seen in parameters when handling was begun and ongoing? How much change in activity was seen? Were there changes in heart or respiration rate or in oxygenation? Did the states vary? How?
3. Were signs of stress seen in the infant? What were they?
4. Did the infant recover control? How long did it take?

After the observation, a case conference should be held to discuss the results and develop appropriate caregiving strategies. For example, if an infant is assessed to be extremely fragile and easily stressed, with little ability to control himself, then interventions incorporating strategies from the areas of environmental modifications, handling, soothing, and positioning to offer a program of *protections* is necessary. The minimal handling protocol would also be imperative (Table 3).

The intervention strategies should be individualized in order to reduce overall activity and handling and protect the infant as much as possible. In addition, methods to provide containment for infants during necessary procedures should be included. Recommendations should be written into the progress notes and nursing care plan and posted at the bedside so that all who interact with the infant (including physicians, respiratory therapists, x-ray technicians, etc.) can participate in the plan. A specific planning session to include the parents' ideas would also be an excellent way to facilitate parent understanding and active participation in meeting the infant's needs.

Reassessment of the behavioral observation should take place at least every week. As the infant progresses, observations can be completed before and after each new transition—for example, when the infant is extubated or moved to an incubator. It cannot be emphasized enough how important *consistency* is to the success of the developmental program. If one shift of nurses is not aware of the plan and does not carry it out, the gains achieved by another shift may be ineffective. Moreover, one cannot underestimate the power of a consistent primary caregiver who can become familiar with the infant's states, reactions, and degree of tolerance over time.

## Intervention Strategies

The goals of developmental care for the BPD infant include promoting weight gain, preserving energy, fostering self-control, reducing agitation, and promoting parent-infant interaction. Strategies to ameliorate stress and disorganization must be based on careful behavioral observation and individualized to the age and clinical condition of the infant. Interventions may be specific to the fragile infant who needs protection from environmental stimuli or to the recovering infant who needs facilitation of appropriate social interaction. Ongoing observation of the infant's responsiveness to interventions is always required. If at any time any activity disturbs an infant, as evidenced by avoidance behaviors, it must be stopped.

Both nonpharmacologic and pharmacologic interventions may be included. However, applying behavioral interventions prior to pharmacologic interventions often prevents stress without the need for medication. The infant's behavior can then emerge into a pattern of autonomous competency rather than chemically mediated coping.

### Strategies for the Fragile Infant

In planning strategies to reduce stress and facilitate central nervous system organization, consider the principles of developmental care.

**Environmental modifications**. Attention to the physical environment around the baby is an important component of developmental care. One may not be able to readily alter the physical environment of the NICU to make it a totally appropriate developmental experience for infants; however, various aspects of this environment can be modified as they affect the infant's experience.

**Facilitation of self-regulation**. Very young babies with BPD may require a complete reduction of stimulation along with interventions that provide the control they need and offer maximal protection from the environment. An example is the minimal handling protocol (Table 3), which has been implemented in some NICUs for infants weighing less than 1,500 gm. As infants mature and can tolerate handling, less protection and more facilitation of attention become the major focus. This emergence of mature control is often *very* gradual in the BPD infant, and episodes of recurring disorganized behavior may still occur.

**Timing interventions**. Ideal intervention strategies will be ineffective and potentially harmful to infants if not appropriately timed. Thoughtful timing of procedures and handling to suit individual infants is fundamental to promoting self-control. Gorski found that timing caregiving procedures to coincide with appropriate infant states produced a positive outcome and that social intervention, inappropriately timed, resulted in signs of distress similar to those following medical interventions.[31] Therefore, overtiring the infant with too much stimulation of any type should be avoided.

**Individualized care**. Infants demonstrate marked variability in their patterns of behavior. They vary in the length and temporal pattern of sleep/wake cycles, activity levels, feeding, and tolerance of visual and auditory input; and they show differences in preference toward stimuli offered by parents.[31] Moreover, what may be an effective intervention one day may not work the next. Flexibility in adapting caregiving to specific infant needs is required to successfully meet the individual infant's specific developmental needs.

**Facilitating interactions.** It is helpful for parents to realize that other developmental needs precede their infant's ability to sustain attention and interaction. This understanding may remedy some parents' eagerness to keep trying to elicit certain responses before their baby is ready to give them. Sensitizing parents to the early stages of behavioral organization, which develop prior to attention, will enhance the chances of a smoother reciprocal relationship and may prevent some of the anxiety and strain parents and staff face when they strive to relate to an unresponsive or agitated infant.

The parents' recognition of their infant's newly emerging, though brief, disorganized alert state can be an emotional moment if they are helped to understand that the infant is trying very hard to get to know them and is acting appropriately for his stage of development. Knowing that their baby cannot sustain or purposefully direct attention at this stage can prevent heightened expectations that lead to disappointing results and leave the parent feeling inadequate, lonely, or resentful.

### Strategies for the Recovering Infant

As infants with BPD develop self-control, they become better able to tolerate several short, routine handling episodes, such as diapering or holding, without excessive fatigue. However, strong stimulation or demanding caregiving activities, such as feeding plus bathing plus dressing, can cause fatigue for many more weeks. The fatigue may be exhibited as mild tachypnea, color change, or exhaustion after feeding or bathing.

When an infant becomes alert and more tolerant to stimuli, he must first master the task of looking *plus* listening and breathing *at the same time.* When he can tolerate more than one activity at a time without disruption of respiration, the infant can probably manage short play periods. However, the length of attention will vary from infant to infant and from day to day, depending on the demands of the infant's daily caregiving and medical regime.

**Enface interaction**. One of the most important developmental activities for the infant is to be able to focus and orient attention to the caregiver's face and to listen. At first, the infant should be presented only with the face to focus on; then the voice may be introduced at a low level. The infant's reactions should be watched closely and the amount and intensity of the face and voice stimulation adjusted accordingly.

**Introducing toys**. As the infant becomes increasingly capable of play without excessive fatigue, an environment that allows him to practice his newly emerging orienting skills can be encouraged. At first, one toy at a time can be placed on the side of the infant's visual field, usually no closer than 8 inches and no farther away than 12 inches. As the infant further develops his ability to stay awake and inspect his surroundings, a mobile can also be offered.

A variety of visually and auditorily interesting colorful toys, offered *one at a time,* will support the infant's ability to focus, follow, and attend. Care should be taken to offer small objects at first, avoiding large, overwhelming toys like huge stuffed animals and dolls. Toys may be colorful. Black, white, or red are more easily seen by neonates, although offering only one or two colors does not encourage visual attention to the full range of visual stimuli available.

Toys with pleasing, soft sounds are also interesting to infants, and they can learn to associate the visual with auditory stimuli. A music box is pleasurable, provided it is not too loud, is of good quality, and is offered at awake periods. A music box may also facilitate transition to sleep states. Sound toys and radios are not useful in the NICU if they only add to the background noise and increase the "white noise" level for the infant. Of course, a parent's voice will be exceptionally pleasing to the infant, and the effect of a parent's voice in promoting attention should not be underestimated.

Caregivers need to monitor the infant closely for the early first signs of fatigue or sensory overload and remove toys or stimuli when these signs are observed. Typical signals include loss of quiet alert state, increased activity, fussing, going to sleep, or gaze aversion. Tachypnea, paling, and loss of tone—particularly in the face—are also common. Attention to each infant's individual signals for rest is imperative to avoid stress and fatigue.

**Creating a learning environment in the crib**. As visual and auditory attention develops, the infant's attention span and responsiveness will increase. When this happens, a mirror can be introduced, so the infant may view himself and his movements. At other times, a dangle toy, such as a small, colorful, soft sounding rattle, can be hung near the infant's hand. As he moves his hands, he may move the rattle, increasing his attention to it as he learns that he made something happen by causing the movement or sound. This experience will induce the infant to repeat the action, touching or moving the toy repeatedly. Placing a small rattle in the infant's hand will facilitate practice of his grasp and visual attention. These activities all must be offered one at a time—and only during the infant's alert, rested, and attentive states.

**Use of infant equipment**. The decision to introduce infant equipment, popular for home use, into the NICU should be carefully considered. First, caregivers must remember that the guidelines for these pieces of equipment are written for full-term healthy infants and do not often provide the same benefit to the sick infant with lung disease. Infant equipment that provides massive amounts of noncontingent stimulation, such as swings, jumpers, and other fast-moving items, should be used judiciously, if at all. The problem is that the infant is unable to control the quality or quantity of stimulation when using such devices.

Equipment that can provide another view of the world and expand the infant's ability to visually inspect his surroundings may be helpful. Infant seats can provide the opportunity to practice visual skills and serve to support the infant in different postures. These seats are recommended for neonates beyond term (corrected age) who can maintain an alert state for at least ten minutes at a time and may be used during feeding of solids or for simply watching the world beyond the crib. We do not recommend that infants sleep in them. Moreover, after 20–30 minutes of sitting in an infant seat, the infant should experience a change in position and either be held or put back in bed. Walkers and high chairs may be used for the infant who has developed head control and some degree of trunk control. Walkers, in particular, provide a rare opportunity for the BPD infant to be upright. The infant must be carefully supported in a proper position and secured safely. Blanket rolls and/or sheets may be used.

It is always important to assess each individual infant's ability to gradually tolerate the new equipment and note his signs for stress and remove him from it *before* excessive fatigue develops. Each piece of equipment must be evaluated as to its value in promoting developmental skills for individual infants based on their ability to tolerate the activity or position. These items should not be used indiscriminately.

**The role of the developmental specialist.** There is an acknowledged need to provide developmentally coordinated care for high-risk infants to improve quality of life. An infant developmental specialist is equipped to respond to that need. Some babies will not benefit from a program of developmental intervention designed to stimulate and encourage responsiveness. If observing and evaluating the infant reveals that he is better organized in a less stimulating environment, the specialist or educator must be willing to request a reduction of activity and a program of protecting the infant. Developmental specialists can also support the staff in managing stress in patients. The specialist's goal should be to help the infant adapt effectively in his current environment.

As the infant matures and develops state control, greater self-regulation, and alerting responses, sensory and movement experiences can be introduced *very slowly* and gradually, always observing the infant's subtle cues so as to facilitate organization responses and avoid disorganization. The developmental specialist can assess early feeding patterns and provide caregivers with appropriate developmental suggestions to assist with nippling. By helping parents understand their infant's behavior or lack of behavior, the specialist can provide parents a caregiving role when they desperately need to be involved with their infant.

The developmental specialist may be a pediatric occupational or physical therapist, an early childhood special educator, a nurse, or a physician. Any developmental specialist providing developmental caregiving in the NICU must become knowledgeable about preterm infant behavior, how to assess that behavior, and how to provide for the unique developmental needs of preterm and sick newborns.

## Pharmacologic Interventions

Sometimes the intervention strategies discussed previously are insufficient to prevent or reduce severe agitation in the BPD infant. Pharmacologic support may be required in those situations to prevent physiologic compromise that may be life threatening or that precludes other treatments. Very little is known about the effects on the developing central nervous system of drugs used for analgesia or sedation. Therefore, the unknown long-term risks of pharmacologic therapy must be weighed against the assessed immediate risks of severe agitation before deciding to use any drug.

The following is a brief review of the medications currently used in the NICU to provide analgesia or to sedate infants.

## Local Anesthesia

The BPD infant is often sensitive to painful stimuli, making it extremely difficult, for example, to obtain a meaningful blood gas from an arterial puncture. The use of a local anesthetic can minimize the pain and subsequent agitation during the procedure. Lidocaine 1 percent (Xylocaine), *without* epinephrine, is the local anesthetic used in the NICU. A small amount (0.05–0.1cc) can be injected subcutaneously at the site immediately prior to the arterial puncture. Lidocaine use should be monitored closely in the infant who is undergoing multiple procedures as it is possible to accumulate significant blood levels with repeated administration. To avoid systemic toxicity, a total amount no more than 0.5 ml/kg of a 1 percent solution should be injected.[32] It has been suggested that a 0.5 percent solution is more appropriate in situations in which repeated injection is required.[33] However, the duration of effect will be shortened (75 instead of 127 minutes in the adult), and more frequent instillation may be required.

The neonate's skin is quite permeable and should provide an effective vehicle for superficial local anesthesia.[34,35] Although the topical application of a lidocaine preparation has provided successful local anesthesia in children, no reports of topical administration of local anesthetics in neonates have appeared in the literature to date.[36,37]

## Nonopioid Analgesics

Nonopioid analgesics alone are effective only against mild pain. They are most effective against pain due to inflammation and are thought to work by inhibition of prostaglandin production. Because of the very serious side effects of salycilates (aspirins), they are not used in newborns.[38]

Acetaminophen has been administered to infants, especially if fever is present. Older BPD infants are especially at risk for upper respiratory and ear infections that are often accompanied by aches, pains, and generalized discomfort, which may present as agitated behavior. Infant metabolism of acetaminophen is poorly understood.[39] Use in children for longer than ten days is not recommended.

Antihistamines have weak analgesic effects but can potentiate the effects of opioid analgesics. The mechanisms of action are not well understood.[40] Hydroxyzine (Vistaril) has been used in pediatrics primarily as a preanesthetic and is not an effective sedative when used alone.[32] Toxic effects and withdrawal symptoms have been reported in neonates with prolonged maternal use of diphenhydramine (Benadryl).[41]

### Opioid Analgesics

Narcotic analgesics are the most powerful drugs available to fight pain. They should always be used with caution, especially in the nonventilated patient because they have the potential to cause histamine release, resulting in some degree of respiratory depression and/or hypotension.[42] Neonates appear to be somewhat more sensitive than adults to the respiratory depressant effects of opioids.[32] These effects are reversible with naloxone (Narcan). Of the narcotics, morphine and meperedine (Demerol) have been most commonly used in infants. There is disagreement as to whether one or the other produces more respiratory depression in the infant. However, the differences between the two drugs may be overestimated. Reaction to opioids is highly individual, and an infant who has an adverse reaction to one agent may be able to tolerate another without problem.

Fentanyl (Sublimaze) is a synthetic opiate often used by anesthesiologists during surgery on neonates.[43–45] Fentanyl is short acting as compared with morphine or meperedine and causes less histamine release and concomitant hypotension.[46] Therefore, it may be more appropriate for use in the BPD infant prior to procedures such as bronchoscopy. High-dose fentanyl is reported to cause muscular rigidity of the trunk area in the adult (stiff-chest syndrome) that can be reversed with pancuronium.[38,47] This side effect has not been reported in infants.[43]

### Sedatives/Hypnotics

Sedatives and hypnotics have no analgesic effects and can even cause a hyperalgic state in which the person has increased sensation of pain.[32] This is important to consider when administering these medications to the BPD infant. If the agitation is the result of pain, a sedative or hypnotic will suppress some of the expression of pain without treating the underlying cause of the agitation. It also may result in excitation rather than sedation. Sedatives and hypnotics are appropriately used for inducing sleep, but they can cause paradoxical reactions in infants and children.

Chloral hydrate is an effective hypnotic for short-term use. It is often the preferred sedative for procedures such as pulmonary function testing or CT scans because it does not affect the central inspiratory drive.[48,49] However, it has been reported that upper airway muscle activity is depressed following chloral hydrate administration, and this may increase the risk of obstructive sleep apnea for some infants.[50] Chloral hydrate is also corrosive to the skin and mucous membranes, and gastric irritation and emesis are not uncommon side effects.[51,52] In addition, it may affect the metabolism of other drugs. An adverse drug reaction between chloral hydrate and furosemide (Lasix), which included symptoms of diaphoresis and variable blood pressure, has been reported in adults.[53]

Because of the very long half-life of chloral hydrate, toxic levels can accumulate with long-term use. Clinical signs of toxicity may manifest as central nervous system and respiratory depression, cardiovascular effects such as arrythmias, and gastric necrosis.[54,55] Use of chloral hydrate for more than seven days should be carefully evaluated, and monitoring of serum levels is suggested.[56] Abruptly discontinuing chloral hydrate can precipitate an acute abstinence syndrome like delirium tremens.[51]

Barbiturates also produce sedation but can cause respiratory depression. Long-acting barbiturates like phenobarbital also have a sedative effect, which diminishes over time and usually disappears within two weeks. Short-acting barbiturates increase risk of producing excitation.[32]

### Anxiolytics

Anti-anxiety agents produce muscle relaxation and calm the patient. These drugs have no analgesic effect and can also produce respiratory depression. As with the sedatives and hypnotics, paradoxical reactions also can occur. Diazepam (Valium) has been used primarily for seizure control in infants. It is effective in calming frantic infants but also has a long half-life and is therefore not suitable for long-term use.

Lorazepam (Ativan) and midazolam (Versed) are short-acting benzodiazepines, similar to diazepam in action. The pharmacokinetics of lorazepam and midazolam in infants and children have not been described. Lorazepam is reported to be successful in controlling seizures in neonates and children and as a sedative prior to pediatric surgery.[57–60] Lorazepam is used in some NICUs for the agitated, hypoxic infant in breaking the cycle of agitation, air hunger, and more agitation. The risk of toxicity with repeated administration is reduced because of its shorter half-life and lack of active metabolites.[61] Because the onset of action when given orally is relatively slow, chloral hydrate is probably a better choice for managing a single acute episode of severe agitation.

### Neuroleptics

The phenothiazines are a class of drugs that produce neuroleptic behavior in adults. These drugs can also potentiate the effects of analgesics and anesthetics. Chlorpromazine (Thorazine) has been reported by some investigators to be relatively safe for newborns.[32] Others advise against its use in infants less than six months of age.[51] Neuroleptic drugs have wide-ranging neurologic and endocrine effects, primarily because of their blockade of dopaminergic pathways. In addition to numerous side effects, these drugs may also be epileptogenic. Therefore, the potential effects of these drugs on the developing central nervous system present some concerns. Chlorpromazine is no longer thought to be useful for treatment of narcotic withdrawal syndrome.[38]

### Physical Dependence Versus Addiction

All psychoactive drugs, including those used to sedate BPD infants, produce some degree of physical dependence and tolerance when given over a period of time. Therefore, dosages should always be tapered before the drug is discontinued. Abruptly discontinuing any psychoactive drug can precipitate withdrawal symptoms because the brain is not able to re-establish neurochemical balance rapidly. The potential for withdrawal symptoms appears to be greater with short-acting rather than longer-acting agents and may occur even at relatively low doses.[61]

The terms "addiction" and "physical dependence" are not synonymous. With addiction, there is a psychological involvement with drug use. It is possible to develop physical dependence without becoming addicted, just as it is possible for the adult to become addicted without becoming physically dependent on the drug.[38] Infants clearly can develop physical dependence to psychoactive drugs, which can be managed by slowly weaning them from the drug. Their capacity for true "addiction" is unknown.

### Selecting an Appropriate Drug

Careful assessment of the infant's condition must precede selection of an appropriate pharmacologic agent. Table 4 lists specific questions to consider before using psychoactive drugs.

If the infant exhibits an acute episode of agitation with severe compromise, such as bronchospasm that is refractory to nonpharmacologic interventions, then immediate use of a drug may be indicated. The agent selected should act rapidly. If the infant has repeated acute episodes over a period of days, scheduled round-the-clock administration of a drug may be indicated. The drug selected should have a relatively short half-life and minimal side effects.

**TABLE 4 ■ Questions To Ask Before Using Psychoactive Drugs**

What behavior is the infant displaying that is actually or potentially harmful?
Is the infant compromised physiologically?
Can any precipitating factors be identified?
Is the oxygen delivery system functioning adequately?
- Is the endotracheal tube properly placed and patent?
- Does the infant need to be suctioned?
- Is the infant's breathing synchronized with ventilator?
- Is increased oxygen necessary?

Have nonpharmacologic comfort measures been attempted?
- Is the infant's temperature stable?
- Has a wet diaper or bedding been removed?
- Has abdominal distention been relieved?
- Has the infant been repositioned, swaddled?
- Has a minimal handling protocol been implemented?

Could the infant be experiencing pain?
- Have procedures been recently performed?
- Have internal sources of discomfort (teething, otitis media, abdominal distress, colic, fractures) been investigated?

What routes are available for delivery of medication?
If sedation alone is required, how long is therapy anticipated to last?
Evaluation of treatment
- Did the drug achieve the desired effect?
- Were there any side effects?
- How will weaning the infant from pharmacologic support be achieved?

Observation of the infant over a period of at least 24 hours, with the infant's state and episodes of compromise recorded, is helpful in determining which drug and dosage schedule are most appropriate. Graphic representation of state and activity may facilitate identification of trends or patterns more clearly than a narrative format.

An infant with BPD in our nursery became increasingly agitated at about three months of age (38 weeks corrected age) despite nonpharmacologic efforts by nurses to modify his environment and reduce his stress. While receiving ventilator support with moderate settings, the infant began to experience periods of severe agitation associated with hypoxemia, copious secretions, and increased airway resistance. Because he could not be adequately ventilated during these episodes, hand ventilation at increased pressures was required. The episodes could sometimes be associated with invasive procedures, but at other times an obvious cause could not be identified.

Chloral hydrate was given during one particularly difficult episode, and the infant relaxed and became easier to ventilate very quickly. However, after one week on a PRN schedule, the nurse noted that the infant was requiring four to six doses of chloral hydrate per day and that the episode of compromise often escalated to a full-blown bronchospasm before the drug would take effect. Because of the concern over potential chloral hydrate toxicity and the desire to prevent rather than simply treat the severe episodes of respiratory compromise, it was decided, during rounds, to administer lorazepam every six hours, even if the infant was not agitated. The purpose was to allow the infant to be relieved of agitation and improve oxygenation. It was hoped that after a week of sedation, the infant's respiratory condition would have stabilized, allowing tolerance of increased activity. The nurses were asked to observe the infant's overall activity level and to monitor closely for any change in the quality or frequency of the agitated episodes.

The infant remained on the round-the-clock sedation schedule for approximately ten days. He also received morphine on four occasions as a premedication prior to procedures. At the end of ten days, significant progress had been made in weaning his ventilator pressure and rate. He was awake for longer periods and could tolerate periods of upset. It was then decided to begin weaning from lorazepam. Decreases in dosage were alternated with increases in the dosing interval until the infant was successfully weaned from the drug over a period of eight days. He still would require an occasional dose of chloral hydrate when his agitation interfered with ventilation, but those episodes decreased as the infant became increasingly able to achieve control with only nonpharmacologic support provided.

## Conclusions

This chapter has illustrated how developmentally appropriate care should be instituted prior to pharmacological intervention in the NICU to reduce BPD infant stress and enhance recovery. Developmentally appropriate care tailored to each infant's individual needs can contribute to improved outcome for infants with BPD. Integration of developmentally appropriate care in the NICU setting requires modification of the infant's immediate physical environment; careful, sensitive observations by staff; modification of routine medical protocols; and most important, modification of knowledge and attitudes of the infants' caregivers.

Caregiving that takes into account each infant's developmental needs is not just an adjunctive therapy requiring simply that another consultant be called in on the case; it requires instead that the professionals who care for high-risk infants have knowledge of neurobehavioral development of preterm and full-term neonates. It requires that caregivers have advanced training in the assessment of infant behavior. It also requires that the knowledge gained from appropriate assessments be used to developmentally support the recovering infant by reducing stress and enhancing self-regulation.

Current theory and research point to a greater impact of daily experience on neurobehavioral development than was previously known. Future research should prove this link even stronger and show the importance of incorporating developmental considerations into every caregiving activity and medical intervention performed in the NICU, thereby improving the developmental outcome of the BPD infant.

## Case Study

Justin C. was born at 28 weeks gestation, weighing 1,000 gm. The first child of a 32 year old mother, he was delivered by emergency cesarean section at a community hospital and transferred to the NICU 28 miles from the parent's home. Justin's progress was characterized by an up and down course, marked by eight weeks on the ventilator, a patent ductus arteriosus ligation, and the development of severe BPD. By the time he was five weeks old, Justin had gained a reputation among the nurses as a difficult baby.

Justin's bed was located in the busiest part of the NICU under a loud speaker system and near a frequently used door. He lay on his back uncovered most of the day so the nurses could see his UA line and was occasionally repositioned on his side. Justin's parents visited three or four times weekly and were afraid to touch him. They sat by the bedside, looking worried, bewildered, and helpless.

When Justin was five weeks old, the nurses observed that he was highly reactive to any touch or handling—especially after procedures such as suctioning or drawing a blood gas. They described his periods of upset as "wild" and stated that he kicked his feet and arms into the air and moved them in all directions. This would be accompanied by arching his head and neck and squirming in a pattern of frantic activity. His face would look as if he were in pain as he grimaced and frowned. After a few minutes of this frantic activity, he would collapse into exhaustion, his color dusky, his respirations suddenly decreased with retractions, and his arms and legs suddenly limp. All movement would cease. He appeared to be asleep, but was actually completely exhausted and unable to move.

The nurses who knew him best were assigned the task of observing and evaluating Justin's behavioral responses. He was determined by all observers to be extremely fragile and easily stressed, and the nurses reported that several handling events could be altered to prevent irritability. The following plan was written up and posted at his bedside with his parents' agreement:

**Justin's Care Plan #1**

1. Environmental modifications:
   Reduce light:
   - Shield head with blanket taped over bed.
   - Remember to shield his eyes when removing blanket or reposition to avoid direct exposure to light.

   Reduce noise:
   - Relocate Justin's bed to a quieter corner of the NICU (away from noise, doors, sinks, overhead speaker).
   - Avoid talking over his bedside.
   - Pad any nearby noisy trash cans or doors.
2. Positioning:
   - Never leave Justin on his back.
   - Position prone and rotate to side lying, changing q 2–4 hours. (*Note:* This may be contrary to unit policy for an infant with a UA line or may require a physician's order.)
   - Encourage flexion; avoid positions that increase limb extension.
   - When turning over or repositioning, turn *slowly,* containing limbs.
   - Position or swaddle, and place rolled blankets at sides and feet.
3. Handling:
   - Adhere to minimal handling protocol.
   - Avoid touch unless absolutely necessary.
   - Before beginning stressful procedures, position with limbs contained (may require second person).
   - Continue to hold limbs during procedure and after; keep holding until Justin is calm, recovered, and able to maintain position by himself (may be up to five minutes). Check heart rate, respiration rate, and oxygen pressure, and stay with him until he is stable.
4. Soothing:
   - Never leave in supine position. Use prone or side lying positions, and cover or lay hands on arms and legs to contain in flexed posture until he is able to remain calm.
   - Remove support *gradually and slowly.*
   - Provide opportunities for nonnutritive sucking.
   - If very agitated, position Justin prone, swaddle, reduce light and noise, give pacifier, and pat gently on back.

At first, Justin's parents were bewildered, but as his nurses gained confidence in managing his stress and preventing his upset, his parents began to recognize Justin's subtle ways of signaling stress. They learned to judge how much energy he had for daily routine events like bathing or diaper change and knew that a sudden drop in respiration rate accompanied by increased paleness were the first signs of his loss of control and probably sensory overload. When they reduced their handling or covered or contained him, he would calm. His parents and nurses continued to offer environmental supports and positioning, and after eight weeks on care plan #1, he no longer needed the interventions for soothing. He wasn't "wild" anymore.

At the end of his fourteenth week of life, Justin was extubated and given a nasal cannula to deliver oxygen by liter flow. He now weighed 2,500 gm and was three and a half months old chronologically, but only two weeks corrected age. At this point, nurses and parents began to note his gradually developing alertness. At first, Justin had opened his eyes and stared ahead for 10–15 seconds, but now he was awake for up to five minutes. His mother, understandably thrilled, wanted to play with Justin. She held him, put her face close to his, and began talking to him with an animated voice, encouraging his attention. Justin reacted by attempting to widen his eyes, but suddenly became pale, tachypneic, then went limp in her arms and became unavailable. (These behaviors were reminders of his old pattern of stress when he had been on the respirator.) Disappointed and frustrated, his mother reluctantly agreed to put him back in his crib, confused that Justin did not seem to want to interact with her.

Justin's nurse, knowledgeable in reactions of premature infants, explained to his mother that Justin had made an impressive effort, but that he wasn't yet sufficiently strong or developed to attend well and coordinate breathing at the same time. She also explained that he was still easily overstimulated. After a brief recovery period in bed, Justin opened his eyes again. Without picking him up, his mother just looked at him quietly. She noticed that when she was quiet and did not talk, he focused on her face for a few seconds, but then looked upset, again rolling his eyes and becoming pale and drowsy. The effort to look seemed at great cost to him, and she felt that she was draining him by asking him to try. His nurse explained that at this stage Justin could handle only one thing at a time and that his patterns of color and respiratory change were the only way he could let his mother know he needed a break. She added that by placing her hands on his feet and holding his hands to contain him and by eliminating attempts to interact, she could help him relax.

At this stage, Justin's care plan was revised to include the following:

### Justin's Care Plan #2

1. Environmental modifications:
   - Maintain previous environmental modifications as well as handling, soothing, and positioning procedures.
2. Facilitating alerting:
   - When he is quiet and alert, hold and cuddle gently.
   - Offer voice *alone or face alone* to support focusing or listening while lying calm in crib.
3. Signs of stress:
   Watch for these signs of stress and if seen, stop activity:
   - Paleness or oxygen desaturation
   - Irregular respirations
   - Limpness of limbs or face
4. To prevent agitation:
   - Carefully plan major caregiving events of the day.
   - Do not bathe, feed, and dress all at once.
   - Give rest periods in between procedures.
5. Feeding routine:
   - Hold and swaddle close to you.
   - Do not look at or talk to Justin during feeds.
   - Let Justin suck on your finger or pacifier to get ready for feeding.
   - Help pace his breathing and feeding efforts by noting when nostrils flare or respiration rate increases above 70 breaths per minute. Then remove nipple, and let Justin regain control of breathing.
   - After feeds, let him rest in prone position with pacifier, swaddled. Remove all toys.

At six months chronological age, three months corrected age, Justin was on cannula oxygen in a large crib. If he was mildly stressed, he would calm himself by sucking on his fingers or pacifier. But if the stress were ongoing (like being suctioned), it required a great deal of effort on his part to remain calm, and Justin would became upset—crying, becoming tachypneic, pale, and fatigued.

He had developed some maneuvers to regulate himself and help his breathing. When placed prone to go to sleep, he would roll halfway onto his side and put his legs together so he could lift his chest partway off the bed. He now gave clear behavioral cues when becoming tired (instead of physiologic cues of color change and respiratory irregularity)—he would yawn, show a tired face, or shift states from quiet alert to active alert or drowsy. He was easily fatigued and had a low energy level and a low threshold for stimulation.

He was always consoled easily when his caregivers recognized his earlier signs of stress and withdrew activities, play, or toys in time for him to calm. He was familiar now with the routine for rest periods, which included being placed prone and covered, given his pacifier, and having the crib covered. When this was employed consistently, he could get to sleep fairly easily and have enough energy for nippling all his feeds. But if too many activities occurred together or he did not get the rest he needed, he grew exhausted quickly and had poor nippling, requiring gavage feeds at night to make up caloric intake.

At this stage, he was functioning between two to four months developmentally in cognitive, social, and fine motor areas. His gross motor and language areas lagged behind at one to two months. His developmental/behavioral care plan was revised to the following:

### Justin's Care Plan #3

For short periods, Justin can tolerate activities and needs to practice them. When he gets tired, showing his stress signals, give him a rest. Activities to encourage include cognitive, fine motor, language, and social skills. When he is alert, rested, and not hungry, play with him.

1. Visual and auditory activities:
    - Help him practice following toys in all directions and turning to their sounds.
    - Talk to him in low tones during caregiving (diapering, etc.).
2. Fine motor activities:
    - Hang one toy at a time (noisy, small, bright) for him to swipe and bat. Remove for naps/sleep.
    - Rotate dangle toys frequently.
    - Let him hold soft, small, cuddly toys with both hands to feel.
3. Social and language activities:
    - Talk face-to-face, letting him lead the "conversation" so he can practice smiling, cooing, and attending.
4. Gross motor activities:
    - A physical therapist will visit daily, and, if Justin is rested and calm, she will help him practice normal movements such as rolling and being held in different positions to facilitate head control.

At all times, Justin needs consistent caregivers who recognize his first signs of stress/fatigue and overstimulation (usually a change from quiet alert to active alert state and an increase in respiratory rate) and who can respond to support his slowly emerging efforts to regulate himself before he loses control, and becomes fussy. He seems to know when he is heading for loss of control and this makes him frantic. He is learning to trust the people who respond to his first signs of stress and help him into calmer situations (such as placing him prone in bed with toys removed and pacifier offered), where he regains control.

His cues for rest are

- moving from quiet alert to drowsy or active alert states
- gaze aversion (looking away from faces or toys and breathing becoming irregular.)

If you do not help him into a calmer situation at *first* sign of these signals, he becomes more and more upset, and it becomes harder to console him. If this happens, these are the situations that help him regain control:

- Place him on tummy with pacifier.
- Cover him with blanket.
- Cover crib so he cannot see out.
- Remove toys from bed.
- Keep bedside quiet.
- Pat his back, but don't look at or talk to him.
- Place his "lovey" (favorite stuffed toy) near him.

Feedings were going well. Some days he could nipple all feeds, but there were other days when he could not finish his feeds and nippled only two-thirds of his required intake. He did best on days he had his primary nurse or mother. Sometimes when he was fed by a nurse who did not know him, he lost his ability to control breathing and feeding earlier in the feed and fed less efficiently. A plan was suggested for these days when calories had to be made up: He was gavage fed at night, and the tube was removed in the morning so nippling could be resumed. He was never pushed; after one or two days, he was usually back on course, nippling feeds.

Now that he could sleep, feed, and play, his parents felt that, even though he was to be discharged while still receiving oxygen by cannula, they had a *real* baby to take home. As discharge approached, Justin demonstrated good neurological and sensory function for an infant who had been hospitalized for seven months and was now four months corrected age. His weight gain was adequate, although he still fatigued easily with new activities. And his parents, feeling more confident now, had learned to watch for his signs of overstimulation and respond accordingly. Moreover, Justin focused and followed his mother's face longer than anyone's and had saved his first smile for her. His mother had also become impressed with the length of time he could now hold a toy, mouth it, look at it, and mouth it again. She had learned that if she gave him a few minutes of quiet time, he could attend quite well to the toy, surprising himself with the movement and sounds he produced.

"We feel we have entered the realm of normal parenting with our child—he is truly blossoming." The best part of this statement by Justin's parents is that it reveals that they knew *they* had played a big role in their baby's development and that they had come through this experience knowing and supporting their baby.

## Behavioral Strategies for the Fragile Infant with BPD

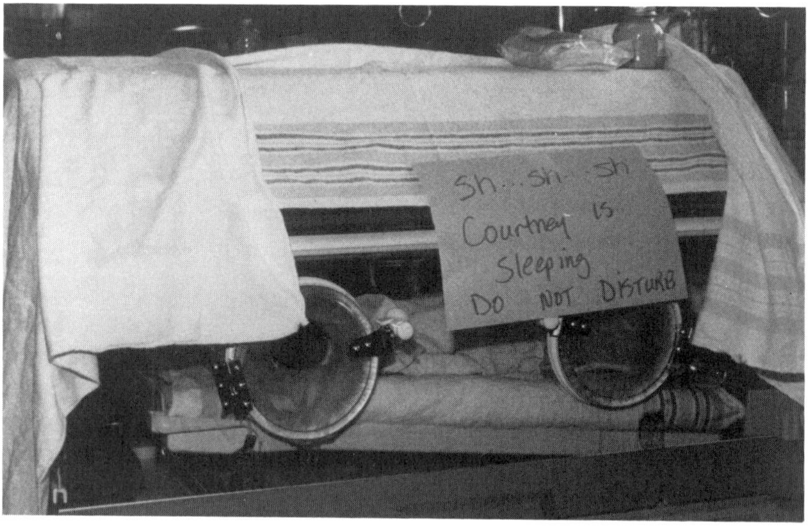


**1. Environmental Protections**

- A "quiet sign" reminds staff and parents to talk quietly away from baby
- Cover overhead lights whenever possible and at night to create day–night cycle
- Place blankets or thick padding on top of incubators to reduce noise inside when bottles, etc. are placed on top (this also shades light)

**2. Handling**

- To prepare infant for stressful procedures, position side lying or prone and offer containment
- Contain during procedures or after taking vital signs
  Complete stressful procedures efficiently, but gently
  Avoid abrupt movements
- Maintain containment and positioning until infant has *completely* calmed

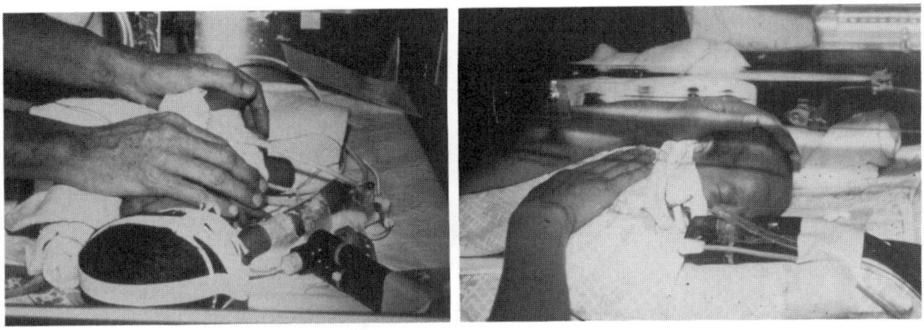

Withdraw support *slowly* (never abruptly)

**3. Positioning**

- Position prone or side lying (avoid supine)
  Cover and swaddle whenever possible
- If you cannot cover or swaddle, position prone or side lying
  Encourage flexion at all times
  Provide props to maintain flexed posture
- Lay four to five thicknesses of blanket under trunk from neck to abdomen to create a pad to curl around
- Positions to *avoid:* supine and flailing
- supine with extended limbs
- supine with hip abduction

**4. Soothing**

- To calm irritability, do *not* pick up an easily stressed BPD infant and talk, hold, rock to soothe; this *adds* to their stress
- Instead, *reduce* activity and handling by placing in bed, prone, cover crib, provide sucking, cover or swaddle, remove toys

**5. Promoting Interactions**

- To prepare for enface interaction:
  Reduce light and noise
  Provide screen for privacy
  Provide necessary supports for alertness (i.e. hand held on chest, hold hands)
  Offer interactions to infant's tolerance level (face alone *or* voice alone at first)
- Infant can maintain alertness for longer than three minutes without significant stress

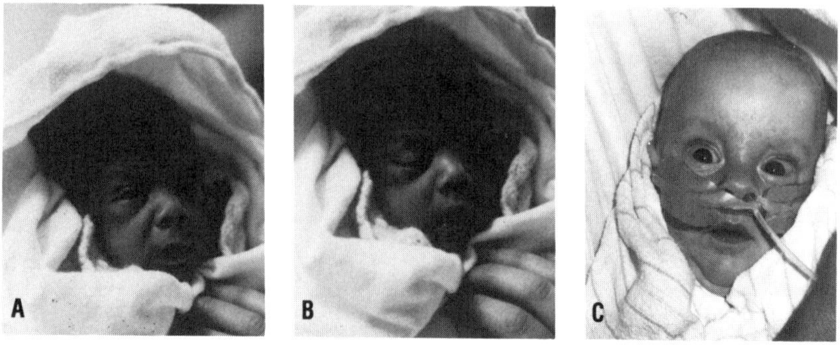


Infant can turn to your voice
Infant can follow your face side to side or fixate on face or scan outer edges
Supports such as pacifier, holding firmly and snugly can help facilitate alerting
Watch for signs of sensory overload

- Know signs of stress or sensory overload
  Facial flaccidity (Photo A)
  Paling or cyanosis
  Irregular respirations or heart rate
  Gaze aversion
  Unavailability—loss of alertness, becoming drowsy, going to sleep, becoming fussy (Photo B)
  Hyperalertness—becoming frantic (Photo C)

## Behavioral Strategies for the Recovering Infant with BPD

### 1. Feeding

- During gavage feedings:
  Time feeding with sleep cycle
  Reduce light and noise
  Avoid social interactions
  Provide containment and support
  Hold if not overly stimulating to infant
  If unable to hold, position side lying on right side, swaddle or cover
  Provide pacifier to suck during nasogastric feedings
- Oral feeding routine:
  Setting the stage:
  Reduce light and noise
  Choose appropriate nipple and test flow through nipple (thicken with rice cereal if flow too fast, causing gulping)

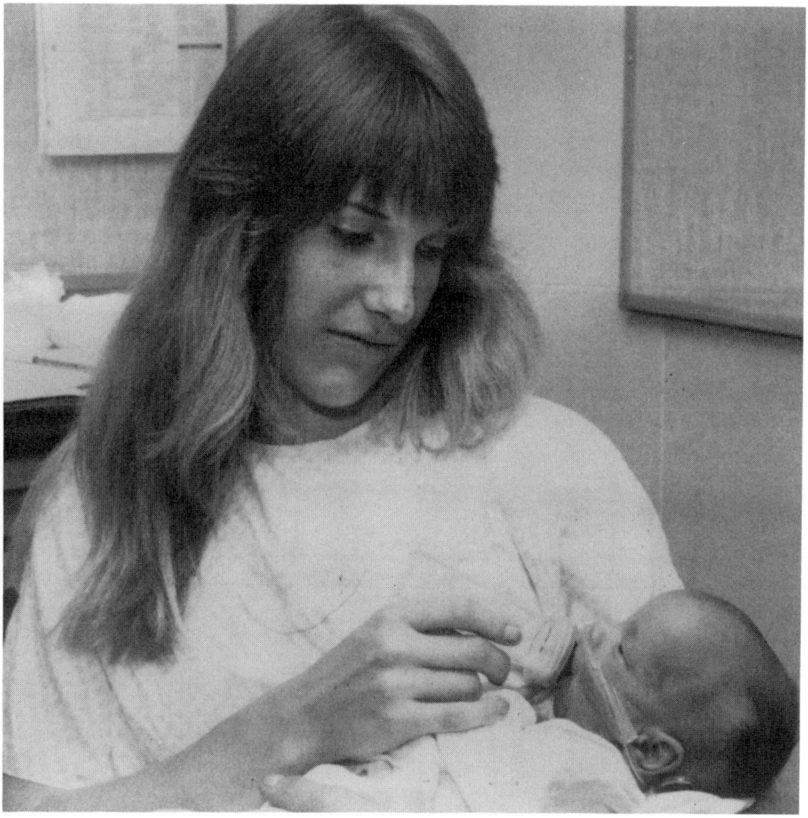

Increase delivered $O_2$ percentage if necessary
The warm up:
Position baby wrapped, flexed, and supported, holding close
Stabilize state (feed in calm alert state).
Assess RR and HR
Note what organizes infant
i.e.: holding hands
providing pacifier first
withdrawing face/voice
offering face/voice
allowing to suck on own hands

- Nippling
  Assess quality and changes in state during nippling
  If able to maintain calm state continue
  Most young BPD babies cannot attend to a face and feed at the same time; They are better coordinated with suck/swallow/breathing, if face and voice are not provided during nippling
- At first sign of stress—if baby becomes stressed with paling, loss of alerting, increase or decrease in RR or HR, remove nipple, and give break. Do not resume until recovered

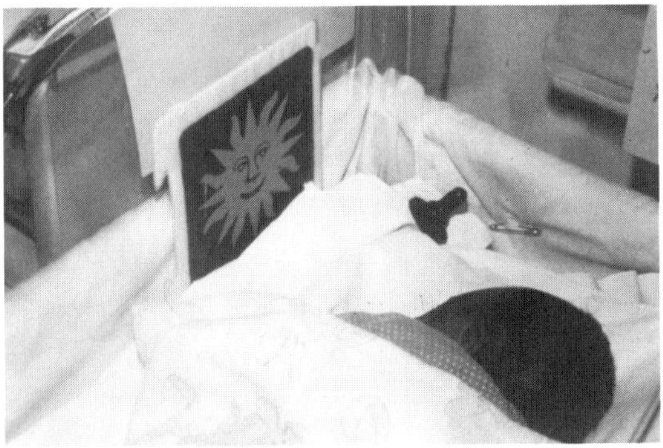

**2. Creating Learning Environment in Crib**

- To encourage alertness and visual attention:
  One clear bright small picture, toy or small mobile can be placed on side of crib
  Remove if infant's stress signals are seen
  A mirror is visually interesting and encourages lengthy visual gazing
  Avoid toys or mobiles that are large and overwhelming
  Remove for sleep if infant cannot calm easily for sleep
- To increase attention and encourage fine motor skills:
  Dangle toys increase attention and ability to bat, grab or reach for toys
  Placing rattles in hand, reaching, encouraging grasp and coordination of touch, visual and auditory attention
- Use of infant seats:
  When positioning infant provide padding and mold to facilitate comfort and good posturing
  Time in infant seat can facilitate alertness; Short periods at first (five minutes) can be lengthened, depending on infant tolerance; NEVER LEAVE INFANT TO SLEEP IN INFANT SEAT

## References

1. Goldson E: Severe bronchopulmonary dysplasia in the very low birthweight infant, Developmental and Behavioral Pediatrics 5(4), 1984, pp. 165–168.

2. Lawson K, Daum CL, and Turkewitz G: Environment characteristics of a neonatal care unit, Child Development 48, 1977, pp. 1633–1639.

3. Gottfried A: The environment of newborn infants in special care units, *in* Gottfried A, and Gaiter JL, eds., Infants' Stress Under Intensive Care, Baltimore, 1985, University Park Press.

4. Gorski PA, Davison MF, and Brazelton TB: Stages of behavioral organization in high risk neonates: Theoretical and clinical considerations, Seminars in Perinatology 3(1), 1979, pp. 61–72.

5. Vohr BR, Bell EF, and Oh W: Infants with BPD: Growth patterns and neurologic and developmental outcome, American Journal of Disabled Children 136(5), 1982, p. 443.

6. Meisels SJ, et al.: Growth and development of preterm infants with RDS and BPD, Pediatrics 77(3), 1986, p. 345.

7. Ruiz MP, et al.: Early development of infants of birth weight less than 1000 grams with reference to mechanical ventilation in the newborn period, Pediatrics 68(3), 1981, p. 330.

8. Fitzhardinge PM, Pape K, and Aistikertis M: Mechanical ventilation of infant less than 1501 grams birth weight: Health, growth and neurological sequelae, Journal of Pediatrics 88, 1976, p. 531.

9. Teberg AJ, et al.: Relationship of prenatal, perinatal and postnatal factors to outcome of infants with birthweights less than 1500 grams, Pediatric Research 14, 1980, pp. 420–439 (abstract).

0. Smyth JA, et al.: Pulmonary function and bronchial hyperreactivity in long term survivors of BPD, Pediatrics 68(3), 1981, pp. 336–340.

1. Franck LS: A national survey of the assessment and treatment of pain and agitation in the neonatal intensive care unit, Journal of Obstetric, Gynecologic, and Neonatal Nursing 16(6), 1987, pp. 387–393.

2. Als H, et al.: Individualized behavioral and environmental care for the VLBW preterm infant at high risk for bronchopulmonary dysplasia: NICU and developmental outcome, Pediatrics 78(6), 1986, pp. 1123–1132.

3. Als H, et al.: Individualized behavioral and environmental care for the VLBW preterm infant at high risk for bronchopulmonary dysplasia and intraventricular hemorrhage, study II: NICU outcome, Abstract: New England Perinatal Association, Woodstock, Vermont, 1988.

4. Als H: Towards a synactive theory of development: Promise for assessment of infant individuality, Infant Mental Health Journal 3(4), 1982, pp. 229–243.

5. Als H: Toward a research instrument for the assessment of preterm infant behavior, *in* Fitzgerald HE, Lester BM, and Yogman MW, eds., Theory and Research in Behavioral Pediatrics, vol. I, New York, 1982, Plenum Press, pp. 35–53.

6. Als H, et al.: Manual for assessment of preterm infant behavior (APIB), *in* Fitzgerald HE, Lester BM, and Yogman MW, eds., Theory and Research in Behavioral Pediatrics, vol. I, New York, 1982, Plenum Press, pp. 65–132.

17. Als H: A synactive model of neonatal behavioral organization: Framework for assessment of the neurobehavioral development in the premature infant and for support of infant's parents in the neonatal intensive care unit, *in* Sweeney JK, ed., The High Risk Neonate: Developmental Therapy Perspectives and Occupational Therapy in Pediatrics, New York, 1986, Haworth Press, 6(3/4) pp. 3–55.

18. Als H, Lester BM, and Brazelton TB: Dynamics of the behavioral organization of the preterm infant: A theoretical perspective, *in* Field TM, et al., eds., Infants Born at Risk, New York, 1979, Spectrum, pp. 173–192.

19. Martin RJ, Okken A, and Rubin D: Arterial oxygen tension during active and quiet sleep in the normal neonate, Journal of Pediatrics 94, 1979, p. 271.

20. Long JG, Philip AGS, and Lucey JF: Excessive handling as a cause of hypoxemia, Pediatrics 65, 1980, pp. 203–207.

21. Long JG, Philip AGS, and Lucey JF: Noise and hypoxemia in the ICN, Pediatrics 65, 1980, pp. 143–145.

22. Burroughs AK, Asonye UO, and Anderson-Shanklin GC: The effect of non-nutritive sucking on transcutaneous $O_2$ tension of non-crying preterm neonates, Research in Nursing and Health 1, 1978, pp. 69–75.

23. Weinstein MR, and Oh W: Oxygen consumption in infants with bronchopulmonary dysplasia, Journal of Pediatrics 99(6), 1981, pp. 958–961.

24. Karp TB, and Harris TR: Neonatal bronchospasm and its complications, Perinatology-Neonatology, May/June 1985, pp. 35–37.

25. Braun MA, and Palmer MM: Early Detection and Treatment of Infants and Young Children with Neuromuscular Disorders, New York, 1982, Therapeutic Media, pp. 54–55.

26. Morris SE: The normal acquisition of feeding skills: Implications for assessment and treatment, *in* Palmer MM, ed., Therapeutic Media, chapter 6, Key issues in the development of abnormal oral moter skills in infancy, New York, 1982, pp. 66–70.

27. Gorski PA, Hole WT, and Leonard CH: Direct computer recording of premature infants and nursery care: Distress following two interventions, Pediatrics 72(2), 1983 pp. 198–202.

28. Lawhon G: Management of stress in premature infants, *in* Angelini DJ, et al., eds. Perinatal/Neonatal Nursing: A Clinical Handbook, Boston, 1986, Blackwell Scientific Publications, pp. 319–328.

29. Brazelton TB: Brazelton Neonatal Assessment Scale, London, 1973, Spastic International Medical Publications.

30. High P, and Gorski PA: Recording environmental influences on infant development in the ICN: Womb for improvement, *in* Gottfried A, and Gaiter JL, eds., Infants' Stress Under Intensive Care, Baltimore, 1985, University Park Press.

31. Gorski PA: Premature infant behavioral and physiological responses to caregiving interactions in the intensive care nursery, presented at First World Congress on Infant Psychiatry, Estoril, Portugal, April 1980.

32. Roberts RJ: Drug Therapy in Infants: Pharmacologic Principles and Clinical Experience Philadelphia, 1984, W.B. Saunders.

33. Bashein G: Use of excessive lidocaine concentrations for local anesthesia, New England Journal of Medicine 302(2), 1980, p. 122.
34. Montagna W, Van Scott E, and Stoughton R: Advances in Biology of the Skin, vol. 12: Pharmacology and the Skin, New York, 1972, Appleton-Century-Crofts.
35. Nachman RL, and Esterly NB: Increased skin permeability in preterm infants, Journal of Pediatrics 79, 1971, pp. 628–632.
36. Hallen B, and Uppfeldt A: Does lidocaine-prilocaine cream permit pain free insertion of IV catheters in children? Anesthesiology 57, 1982, pp. 340–342.
37. Tree-Trakarn T , and Pirayavaraporn S: Postoperative pain relief for circumcision in children: Comparison among morphine, nerve block, and topical analgesia, Anesthesiology 62(4), 1985, pp. 519–522.
38. Gilman AG, Goodman LS, and Gilman A, eds.: Goodman and Gilman's Pharmacologic Basis of Therapeutics, New York, 1980, Macmillan.
39. Peterson P, and Rumack B: Pharmacokinetics of acetaminophen in children, Pediatrics 62, 1978, pp. 877–879.
40. Rumore MM, and Schlichting DA: Clinical efficacy of antihistamines as analgesics, Pain 25, 1986, pp. 7–22.
41. Parkin DE: Probable benadryl withdrawal manifestations in a newborn infant, Journal of Pediatrics 85(4), 1984, p. 580.
42. Mather LE, and Phillips GD: Opioids and adjuvants: Principles of use, *in* Cousins MJ, and Phillips GD, eds., Acute Pain Management, New York, 1986, Churchill Livingstone.
43. Robinson S, and Gregory GA: Fentanyl-air-oxygen anesthesia for ligation of patent ductus arteriosus in preterm infants, Anesthesia Analgesia 60, 1981, pp. 331–334.
44. Yaster M: The dose response of fentanyl in neonatal surgery, Anesthesiology 63(3a), 1985, p. A471.
45. Hickey PR, et al.: Pulmonary and systemic hemodynamic response to fentanyl in infants, Anesthesia Analgesia, 64, 1985, pp. 483–486.
46. Rosow CE, et al.: Histamine release during morphine and fentanyl anesthesia, Anesthesiology 56, 1982, pp. 93–96.
47. Christian CM, Waller JL, and Moldenhauer CC: Postoperative rigidity following fentanyl anesthesia, Anesthesiology 58(3), 1983, pp. 275–277.
48. Hunt CE, Hazinski TA, and Gora P: Experimental effects of chloral hydrate on ventilatory response to hypoxia and hypercarbia, Pediatric Research 16, 1982, pp. 79–81.
49. Lees MH, et al.: Chloral hydrate and the carbon dioxide chemoreceptor response: A study of puppies and infants, Pediatrics 70(3), 1982, pp. 447–450.
50. Hershenson M, et al.: The effects of chloral hydrate on genioglossus and diaphragmatic activity, Pediatric Research 18(6), 1984, pp. 516–519.
51. Martindale: The Extra Pharmacopeia, 27th ed., London, 1978, Pharmaceutical Press.
52. Kuzemko JA, and Hartley S: Treatment of cerebral irritation in the newborn: Double-blind trial with chloral hydrate and diazepam, Developmental Medicine and Child Neurology 14, 1972, pp. 740–746.

53. Malach M, and Berman N: Furosemide and chloral hydrate: Adverse drug reaction, Journal of the American Medical Association 232(6), 1975, pp. 638–639.
54. Laptook AR, and Rosenfeld CR: Chloral hydrate toxicity in a preterm infant, Pediatric Pharmacology 4, 1984, pp. 161–165.
55. Nordenberg A, Delisle G, and Izukawa T· Cardiac arrhythmia in a child due to chloral hydrate ingestion, Pediatrics 47, 1971, pp 134–135.
56. Hartley S, Franck LS, and Lundergan F: Maintenance sedation of agitated infants in the NICU with chloral hydrate: New concerns, Journal of Perinatology 9(2), 162–164.
57. Deshmukh A, et al.: Lorazepam in the treatment of refractory neonatal seizures: A pilot study, American Journal of Diseases in Children vol. 140, 1986, pp. 1042–1044.
58. Lacey DJ, et al.: Lorazepam therapy of status epilepticus in children and adolescents, Journal of Pediatrics 108(5), 1986, pp. 771–774.
59. Burtles R, and Ashley B: Lorazepam in children, British Journal of Anesthesia 55, 1983, pp. 275–278.
60. Kyriakopoulos AA, Greenblatt DJ, and Shader RL: Clinical pharmacokinetics of lorazepam: A review, Journal of Clinical Psychiatry 34(10-2), 1978, pp. 16–23.
61. Perry PJ, and Alexander B: Sedative/hypnotic dependence: Patient stabilization, tolerance testing and withdrawal, Drug Intelligence and Clinical Pharmacy 20, 1986, pp. 532–537.

## CHAPTER 7

# The Family of the Infant with Chronic Lung Disease

*Donna Carson, MSW, MED*
*Emory Regional Perinatal Center*
*Emory School of Medicine, Department of Pediatrics*
*Atlanta, Georgia*

With the advent of modern neonatal nurseries, we have witnessed many miracles as the number of infants who survive has increased dramatically. We have also seen a different type of patient—the infant with chronic lung disease who will remain in the hospital many months after his birth. These patients do not fit in the traditional pediatric population, yet they differ from the usual premature infant in the neonatal unit. They present dilemmas for the NICU staff who are often unaccustomed to these "older" children, and they create even more difficulties for the parents who must continue to await their child's homecoming. How do the families of these "high-tech survivors" cope with the long wait, the frequent changes in condition, the never certain outcome, and the physical, emotional, and financial stresses that they must deal with? How can we best help them endure, cope, participate, and remain a family?

Families of babies placed in the NICU enter a strange new world, one for which few are prepared. The sights and sounds of the nursery with all its unfamiliar and high-tech equipment are enough to traumatize anyone, but to have one's own child as an appendage of that equipment is truly overwhelming.

Immediately, the parents must begin to deal with the realities of a premature or sick infant: the uncertainty of survival, the lack of predictability of outcome, and a sense of failure, loss, anger, and guilt. These feelings are intensified when the infant must be transported to another facility, and separation is added to the other issues that confront the parents. The entire process of normal bonding between infant and family is threatened by the birth of a sick newborn.

For the first few days in particular, the focus of the family and staff is generally on whether or not the infant will survive. Parents are usually so focused on this point that they may not clearly hear or absorb the words, "The ventilator can also damage the lungs." During this early critical period, making it through another day without seeing an acute deterioration in their child is their measure of success.

But as these days add up, everyone begins to understand that this child will not be ready for discharge "about when he should have been born." Rather, his lung disease will mandate that he remain in the nursery for many months. Many parents suggest that this becomes a reality for them when their child is about three months of age. By this time, they have seen many other infants who started out like their own come and go—yet theirs remains ventilator dependent, making slow progress, if any.

Miller has identified three stages of parental adaptation: (1) disintegration (most clearly represented by shock, denial, and disbelief), (2) adjustment (shown by anger, bitterness, grief, mourning, despair, guilt, rejection, and attempting to restore some kind of balance to their lives), and (3) reintegration or acceptance of the child and situation.[1] However, rather than being able to progress through the stages of adaptation, the family of an infant with chronic lung disease is often stuck in a situation of chronic grief—the situation doesn't have a point of resolution but continues on and on. This places families of infants with chronic lung disease or other illnesses requiring long, unstable hospital courses in a particularly vulnerable emotional situation. Their initial coping strategies may have worked well, but the extended period of crisis has stressed both the family and their social support systems to the limits.

Parents often relate just how difficult it is for them to feel like they are parents and really attached to their infant who has never been home with them. They mention feeling that the baby is not really theirs but is more or less "on layaway." It is difficult to find a role as a parent because of the infant's medical limitations, nursery rules and regulations, the fear, and the "unrealness" of the entire situation. Constantly living in fear that the child might never go home, many parents make a deliberate decision as to whether or not to get involved with and attached to their baby.

All parents look for comparisons and points of reference when their baby is first born. They see babies in the crib or isolette next to their baby's: some of them make it and leave the NICU, others die. Parents begin to look around for other babies whose condition, appearance, and equipment seems the same as their own child's; then they inquire about that child's status. If the object of comparison has done well, it gives the parents hope; if the child is more chronic, it can prepare the parents for a long and similar course.

They look to the staff for the subtle cues and words that will either give them hope for their child's survival or help them remain a bit aloof and detached. Always present is the knowledge that at any moment the situation can change drastically—that death is a very real possibility. Parents ask the staff, "Have you ever had any baby like this survive?" to try to get a feel for what they need to prepare themselves for.

Staff do not like to compare one baby with another, so they may try to guide parents away from making these comparisons. Yet parents desperately need to have something concrete to hang onto. Perhaps that is why weight gain often remains a primary concern for parents—even when everything else has gone wrong.

Because most parents do not have previous experience with an intensive care nursery, they do not initially know what to ask and what to expect. In time, they learn what questions to ask, they find out what is permissible for them to do, and they begin developing their own system of coping.

Among the variable factors that can impact a family's ability to cope and adapt are age, educational level, temperament, the presence and strength of relationships with significant others, occupation, health, values, meaning of the pregnancy and child, financial situation, life situation, previous experiences with crises, cultural and religious background, and extended family and community support. All these factors individually and jointly affect how staff and family interact and how the family copes with the crisis of a sick child.

The greater the number of negative factors in operation for a given family, the more necessary is intervention by the nursery staff to address specific problem areas and determine helpful strategies. For example, the very young teenage mother, not thrilled about her pregnancy to begin with, who delivers a premature infant requiring maximum care is at a high risk for not bonding with the infant, not ever becoming involved in the care, and being "lost" to the staff and child. The staff often become angry in this situation as they feel they are put in the position of having to "sell" the baby to the parents. If they aren't effective, however, they end up with an infant who has no one because the parent was lost early on.

When the infant's condition seems time-limited, the staff and the family are usually able to tolerate the situation and each other, knowing that this will not go on forever. When the infant's condition evolves into one like chronic lung disease with a prolonged hospitalization, the family and staff often have problems coping with each other, as well as with the infant. If the working relationship between staff and family becomes disrupted, it is detrimental to all parties involved. Families are labeled "difficult," and staff may request that they not care for that particular infant. Staff contact with parents may be strained or even avoided, and the parents may be excluded from the NICU or certain aspects of care. All this may alter the delicate parent-infant relationship that is developing at a very important time for both parent and infant.[2] Competition between parents and nurses has been described and can subtly undermine the situation further.[3]

The following case studies are of two mothers who had infants hospitalized for long periods after birth due to chronic lung disease. They reflect different coping styles and point out various problems and solutions encountered by staff and parents.

### Case Study 1

Mr. and Mrs. S. were in their mid thirties, the parents of three children, ages 10, 8, and 4. They had experienced a late miscarriage two years before Jacob's birth. Mrs. S. needed a circlage, had premature rupture of membranes at 27 weeks, and was referred to a regional perinatal center 60 miles from home for management. Jacob was born at 27 weeks gestation weighing 800 grams. He was intubated and, because of lack of staffing and bed space, was immediately transported to another facility 70 miles away from the regional center. Excerpts from a taped interview with these parents reveal the difficulties they had in getting involved in his care and coping with the situation.

*Mrs. S*: "I don't know if I felt really attached to Jacob at first. He was taken so quickly; I just saw something blue pass by. His father went with him to the other hospital and felt hopeful because there was another baby there about Jacob's size who was doing pretty well. That made us feel like there was hope for our baby; we began to feel he was going to live.

"He stayed in that nursery for the next two months, but *I never really felt bonded* to him because we just didn't get to spend much time with him because of the distance. He was also so fragile and had so much equipment that *we didn't want to bother him.*"

*Mr. S*: "Of course I never felt he was like one of my other children because he was so far from home. It was a while before I felt he was really ours. We were told early on that he had chronic lung disease and would be in the hospital 'a long time,' but we never really understood what that meant.

"We got that book by Helen Harrison (*The Premature Baby Book*).[4] That helped us understand some things and to hang on to hope. We kept thinking that once he got to be five pounds, he could come home. Somehow we just didn't focus on the lungs but were more concerned with his weight.

"At first we just kind of believed everything the doctors said. We hated to take up their time, so the nurses answered most of our questions. After a while it seemed like every doctor was doing something different. Both of us got to where we would question them. I think one of the hardest things was the doctors changing every month. Each new doctor would come in with a new idea to try on Jacob."

*Mrs. S*: "The *lack of privacy* was also a real problem for us. You always felt that you had to do what everybody else was doing. I was afraid to pinch his cheeks or undress him or talk babytalk to him—there were always so many people around.

"Some of the things that helped at first were really special. The nurses would write letters to us from Jacob, make cute name tags for his bed every week; they left me a rose on Mother's Day from him, and even called me so I could hear the noise he made breathing the day he was weaned off the ventilator. They really made me feel like I had a baby, and I appreciated all the trouble they went to. I've kept all those letters in a scrapbook.

"We *wanted* the nurses to get attached to him so that they would make sure he got good care when we weren't there. When he got a foster grandmother and volunteers, that helped, too. We wanted him to be loved and held as much as possible.

"I had to make a decision about being at home with my family or being with Jacob. I usually went up a couple times during the week and tried to make the trips fun for the kids. They loved coming to see Jacob, and they went through all the hurts, too. They knew when we were upset, and we tried to deal with it as a family. I think that the experience actually strengthened our family. The time driving 60 miles to and from the hospital gave us the opportunity to talk to each other and stay in touch with how we were doing. Even crying on our way back from the hospital let us unwind, get our feelings out, and try to understand what was going on. We'd also think of the questions we wanted to ask when we got there and just try to get prepared for the ups and downs. But I don't think we were ever really ready for any downs.

"We would call ahead and think he was doing great, and by the time we got there, he'd be bruised all over or running a fever, or they couldn't get an IV in. *That* was traumatic for me. There were many times when I felt I just couldn't make it when I saw Jacob like that. That was hard, you know, emotionally. Our religious faith really helped us get through most of the time. I just felt so helpless seeing him on the brink—hurting and slipping and nobody able to calm him down —or when they couldn't find a vein, and he was covered in bruises. And all of those x-rays! I thought if he didn't die from lung problems, he'd die from cancer. But this was all we knew to do for him."

*Mr. S:* "There were so many people. We would call and not know who his nurse was. That was hard. I knew there were certain nurses who loved him and would check on him when we weren't there; we relied on some of the other babies' mothers to check on him, too."

*Mrs. S:* "When he was in the intermediate level, he was managed by nurse practitioners. We loved that. They were all so practical and down to earth and seemed to spend more time with him. I felt so comfortable just calling them and saying, 'Hey, what's going on?' They always made us feel like he really was our son. I'd watch the nurses with the other babies and decide, 'That's the one I want for Jacob.'"

At many points during his stay, Jacob seemed to be nearing the time when he might be discharged home on oxygen. Each time, he seemed to slide backward, and the decision was delayed. He acutely deteriorated at seven months of age and died unexpectedly. His parents took him home in their car to arrange his burial.

*Mrs. S*: "I never expected him to die. I just kept waiting for him to get better and felt he was safe since he had made it so far. He had looked so good that day. We just weren't ready."

*Mr. S*: "After he died, I just wanted to take him home without all that stuff on him—just to be with my son and take him home. We finally had some time for our family to be together. We saw a lot of good things that came out of Jacob's life: We're thankful for what we have; we're thankful for the time we had to know him and for all the lives he touched. We still look at all of the letters and pictures and miss him. Our kids still talk about him and miss him, too."

This family's story is fairly representative of what goes on during a chronic hospitalization. The issues they raise are the critical ones that NICU staff must be attentive to because they reflect what the family has to deal with in addition to the child's illness.

### Case Study 2

Rachel was a term infant hospitalized for 21 months from birth. This was the first pregnancy for her mother; her father had a seven-year-old daughter

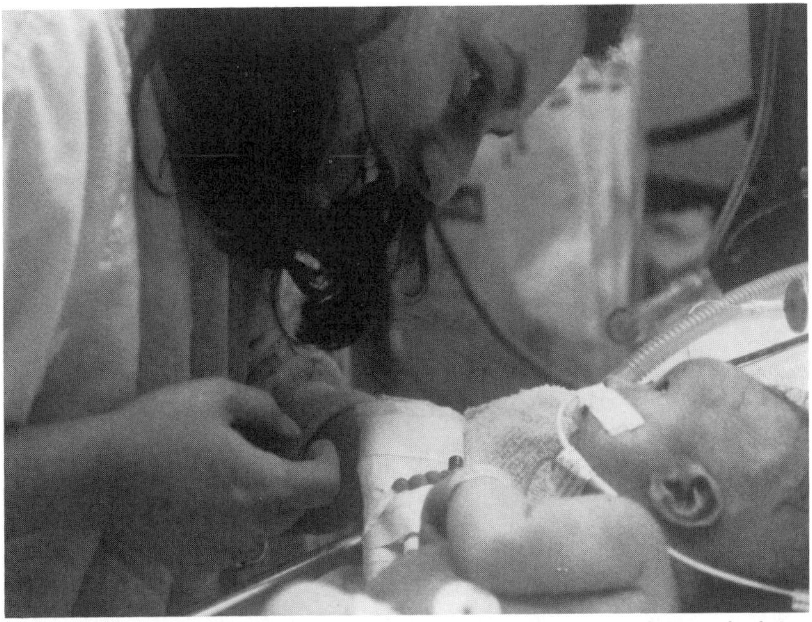

***Rachel and mother at one month: "At the beginning I didn't really feel like she was mine but that she belonged to the hospital."***

by a previous marriage. Rachel was born with a relatively rare condition known as pentology of Cantrell, consisting of five major defects: omphalocele, short sternum, ventricular septal defect, incomplete rib cage, and small lungs. She required surgery immediately after birth and five more times during the first six months of life, including open heart surgery. She developed chronic lung disease.

The words of Rachel's mother reflect the stresses and adaptations that parents of a baby with chronic lung disease experience during prolonged hospitalization:

"Rachel was transported out to the children's hospital in our town immediately after birth. Her problems were totally unexpected. Since her diagnosis was rare, no one could predict her outcome or the course; no one could really tell us anything other than she would be in for a long, long time and would need several surgeries. It was months before I realized how sick she was. All I kept wanting was for her to come home. Whether she would even survive was in question; during open heart surgery they almost lost her.

"I thought long term was a few months—not 21 months. I realized after about 5 or 6 months that I just needed to hope for the best and take one day at

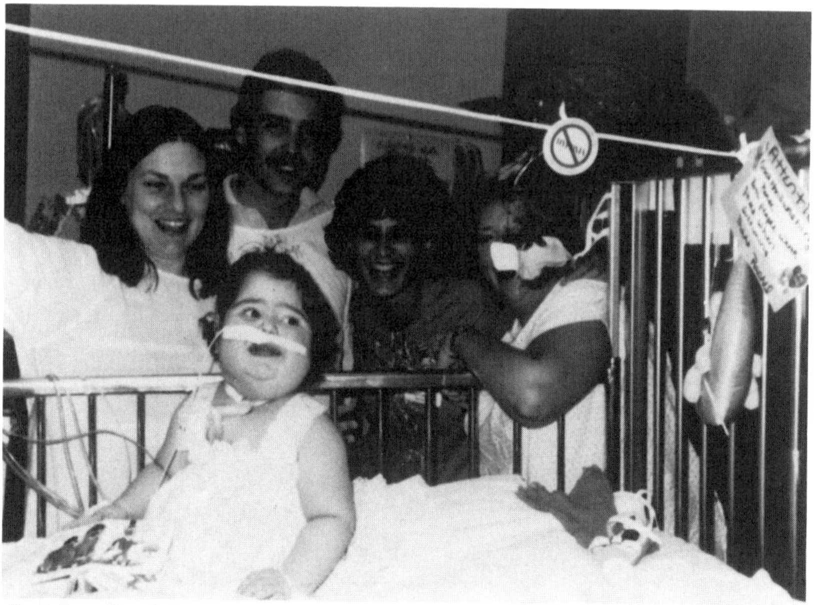

***Rachel, mother, father, and primary nurses: "Rachel had her own core of nurses along with her primary nurse; they knew her likes and dislikes, and we knew them."***

a time instead of always looking to the future and hoping she was going to come home. I slowed myself down a little bit and thought, 'What happens happens.'

"At the beginning, I didn't really feel like she was mine but that she belonged to the hospital—a guinea pig and part of a guessing game. When she was a month old, I was able to hold her. They had just started a normalization program. It was an attempt to make her life and ours (and other kids who were in the hospital a long time) more normal. In the beginning, some nurses would say, 'When I get time, I'll get her up.' In the normalization program, they really stressed to the nurses that it was important for the parents to hold their child and to get involved. At six weeks I started giving her sponge baths and bringing her ribbons for her hair and clothes. I had to remember all of her equipment when I went shopping, looking for things with elastic to go over arm boards. It was bad when friends would buy Rachel clothes; I'd open the box, look at it, and say, 'It's lovely, but...she can't get that over her IV. Do you mind if I return it?'

"I went to the hospital daily for eight hours a day. My husband came almost every day after work. He was really good about understanding my wanting to be with Rachel. We took two vacations during those 21 months, once to Florida and one time to the lake camping. The lake was so close that I jumped in the car and drove to the hospital to see her, leaving my husband sitting in the boat. It was real hard on him because he ended up having to do a lot around the house with my being gone so much.

"I really had a hard time at first. I didn't realize they changed doctors every month; her condition was so rocky, and I felt so stupid, not knowing what to ask or do. I had never been around a sick person. Sometimes I felt the doctors thought I was just another dumb parent. I felt there was little consistency in her care and had a hard time developing trust.

"Then there was one doctor who came on when Rachel was three months. She showed a real interest in Rachel and spent a lot of time explaining things to me and just seeing how I was doing. I asked Rachel's primary nurse if that doctor could be Rachel's primary doctor, and that was finally agreed upon. Even though other doctors took care of her, this doctor managed her overall care and was responsible for her. Before that, we often felt like we were on a roller coaster. I thank God for that doctor every night; she was always there for Rachel and for us—and she made all the difference.

"Rachel had her own core of nurses along with her primary nurse; they knew her likes and dislikes, and we knew them. It was always hard when she sometimes had a nurse from another area who didn't know Rachel or us—we just never felt as comfortable. The primary nurse would set up monthly meetings with the physician, dietician, and physical and respiratory therapists to plan the course for the next month. I later got to attend these meetings and be part of the planning. That really helped. Nobody ever gave up on her.

"We never had any privacy with Rachel. It bothered my husband more than me because he felt uncomfortable being around all the nurses. I would just crawl up in the bed with Rachel and didn't really mind anybody. Her stepsister did fine at first but then went through a period when she didn't want to go see Rachel. I think she was jealous and resented the world revolving around Rachel. I never pushed her, and she later started going again.

"I had a hard time dealing with the rigid rules they had. They wanted me to leave during social service rounds, physician rounds, etc. They felt it was better for me not to be there so much; they thought I was spending too much time there. I was told that it 'wasn't good for me,' and I 'needed to go on with my life.' They couldn't understand that I couldn't do that. The happiest place I was was being in that unit with her. I'd come home at night, and I was miserable. In two hours I was on the phone checking on her. I slept fine, but probably because I was so exhausted.

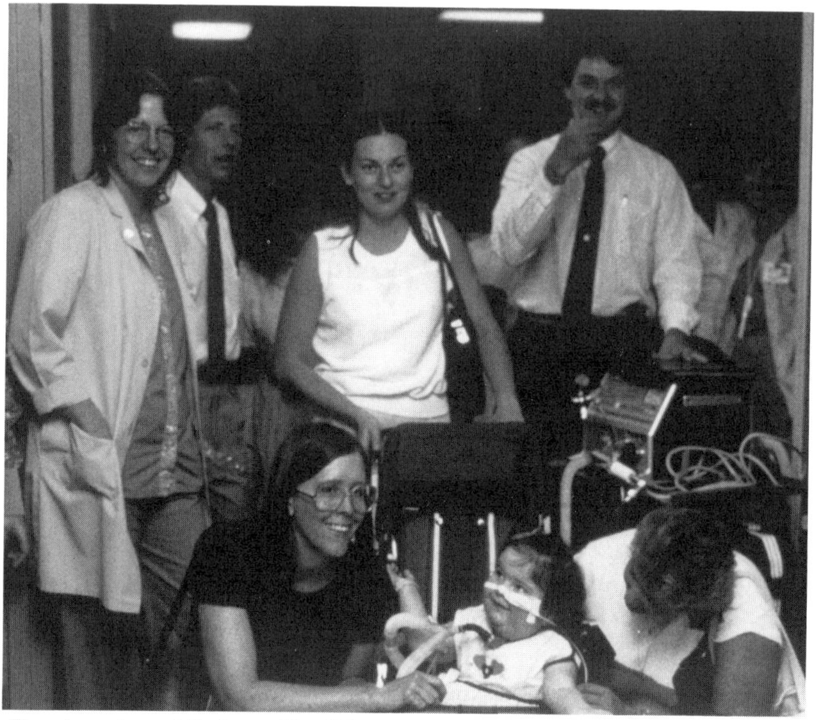

***The primary team at discharge: "Our little team, the primary neonatologist, nurse, physical therapist, and respiratory therapist, had monthly planning meetings and would set goals."***

"I fell apart when they *asked me to stay out of the unit.* She was six months old and more stable, and I felt more confident with her. I cried for eight straight hours. Some of the nurses really pushed for me, especially the nurses who were mothers—they saw that it was good for me and Rachel for me to be there. It finally got to be okay, and they ended up treating me like one of the staff. I needed to be there as a mother and as an advocate. Sometimes they would do things that just didn't seem necessary, and I could at least ask them not to, and that might make things easier on Rachel. I learned what to ask and what to expect; I didn't know either at first.

"Sometimes they said I was good for some of the other moms who weren't so involved and were afraid of their children. They would see me with Rachel and get more involved with their own babies. It seemed like every time I got to be friends with other parents, their baby would die, and that really got to be hard. I also rocked a lot of babies in the unit whose parents lived away.

One little boy's mom was relieved when I rocked him, especially when he moved to the floor. You know they aren't watched as closely once they don't need to be in the unit. He had been in the unit for seven months, so his mom didn't know any of the nurses on the floor. Eventually, I had to stop rocking them because I was getting too close, and some of those kids died. Rachel was enough to deal with.

"It used to be real hard on me to watch all those little premies go home: They weighed a pound and were making progress, and then here was big ol' Rachel. I used to say, 'Come on Rachel, if those kids can breathe, you can do it, too.' I really didn't know whether she'd make it or not until she was *more than a year* old. She's a survivor—she came through everything.

"Our little team, the primary neonatologist, nurse, physical therapist, and respiratory therapist, had monthly planning meetings and would set goals. The staff always decorated her bed on special occasions, dressed her up. They even started a diary for her and wrote the good and the not-so-good things. That was really nice because I read what went on if I ever had to miss a day. I really counted on the staff to be there for me as well as for Rachel. It got difficult always having new people come on each month. I got tired of answering the same questions and orienting people. So I mostly dealt with our own team. The big turnover in nurses was also hard—and over two years, there was a big turnover.

"When Rachel was trached, things got a lot better because then I could get her up and move around without always having to ask permission. She really became more my daughter then. It got to the point where she was medically pretty stable—no IVs, just a ventilator and medicines—and I figured I could do all of that at home. It took many months to get it all worked out with many people helping—special Medicaid waivers, home service companies—and there was so much to learn. I was so glad that after she had been trached, the nurses had taught me how to suction her and do everything, so I had had months to practice. I would have been scared to death if I had learned right before taking her home.

"I'm glad we did what we did now. But during some rocky days, I wondered why we were doing all of this. One day when Rachel had a bad day, I came home and said to my husband, 'I wish she would die.' That upset him terribly, and he sat down and cried. He was very upset at me and asked me never to say that again. The mom of a little boy I rocked said that she had said the same thing and had a hard time admitting that she had those thoughts.

"It *really helped to have someone who didn't take care of Rachel to talk to.* The surgical clinical specialist was an enormous support for me. My church really offered no support, so the people at the hospital and my mother were

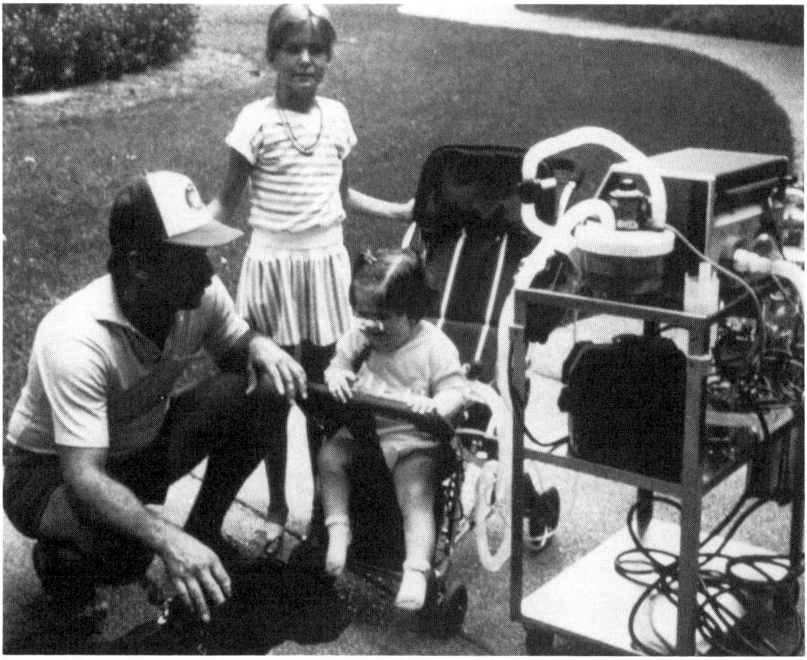

*Rachel, father, and stepsister with family dog in the hospital garden: "When Rachel was trached, things got a lot better because then I could get her up and move around without having to ask permission. She really became more my daughter then."*

our main friends. Money was a big concern, and we were initially upset that the business office insisted we apply for all of these programs on Rachel's second day of life when we didn't even know what was going to happen. Now I'm glad they did.

"If somebody had told me three years ago that this was what I was going to go through, I would have said, 'No way.' Rachel has been the one who has kept me going. She was always alert and really had a personality. She's the happiest child I've ever seen in my life. Nothing gets her down. I'll admit that she's spoiled rotten. Everyone in that hospital knew her, and I really think that helped her make it through. She has taught me a lot, and I feel she's here for a reason. She has taught me patience. As a child, you're taught to care about things and to care about people; then as you grow older, you're just more concerned about yourself. Rachel made me have to sit down and think. I do need to care about other people and other things—and life is very precious, every moment of it."

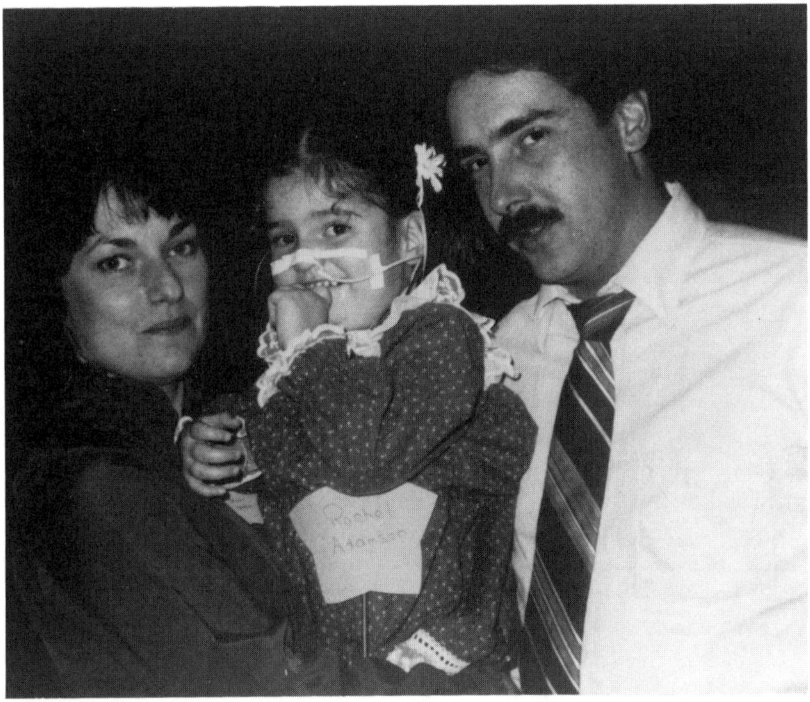

*Rachel, mother, and father at first Christmas at home: "...and life is very precious, every moment of it."*

Rachel has now been home on a ventilator six months; she is off the ventilator 40 minutes a day, and her parents continue to be amazed by her. Her primary nurse is still able to care for her at times, and her primary physician still checks on her at home.

## The Needs of Parents

The stories of these two families point to a number of basic needs that all parents of infants in an NICU have in common, but especially those with a chronically ill infant.

### The Need for Information

Parents look to all levels of staff for information and clarification from the very beginning of the hospitalization throughout the entire experience. For most parents, the need to know what is going on with their child is essential to their being able to learn how to cope with the situation. The explanations may need to be repeated numerous times early on because of the shock the parents are in. They often feel ashamed to ask questions for fear of appearing "dumb" to the staff. With physicians particularly, many parents are reluctant to "take up their time" with questions.

Many parents turn to books for more detailed explanations of what they are encountering. The nursery should either provide a bibliography of helpful books or have a library where parents can read what they wish. It is always wise to caution parents that they will read much that doesn't pertain to their child, and they should try not to generalize the information to their own situation. Often parents begin to feel more comfortable, knowledgeable, and confident in asking questions of the staff after they have read some information about the disease process. This may become uncomfortable for the staff, who are sometimes defensive when questioned directly about procedures, techniques, and so forth. Rather than allowing themselves to become threatened and turn away from the questioning family, the staff should try to honor the family's need to know as an effort to help their child and to regain some degree of control over feeling so helpless and left out.

Sometimes parents are able to obtain information and support from other parents who have had similar experiences. Again, parents must be able to individualize their own experience and acknowledge the differences between their own infant and the other family's infant.

In many situations, parents must rely on the telephone as their primary means of obtaining information about their infant, particularly when the infant has been moved to another city. It is essential that the staff learn how to provide both information and sensitive listening when talking on the phone to these "removed" parents. It is important to talk about more than oxygen level and weight. Describing the child's behavioral activities helps establish his personality to the absent parent. Giving parents the message that their baby is a real person who may smile, cry, wiggle around, and do other "baby things," and not just an attachment to a machine, goes a long way in developing both their relationship with their child and their trust in the caretakers.

### The Need to Feel Like a Parent

The helplessness that parents with a sick infant feel, coupled with the sense of intimidation because the baby is hospitalized, makes feeling like a parent and performing parental activities difficult at best. The staff needs to ensure that parents are consistently involved in decision making about their child—and to be constantly in search of activities that parents can participate in with their child. Simple activities like washing the child's clothes, being able to give the daily bath, dress, and interact with the child—without always having to ask permission—can help the parent feel more involved and lessen the hostile emotions that can emerge when parents feel they have no control over what they are able to do for their child. Learning some of the care needs—suctioning, aerosols, chest PT—can not only help the parent participate in the child's care in the hospital, but also lessen the fright they are likely to feel if this level of care is required later at home. There must be a willingness on the family's part to share their child with the staff and of the staff to share the infant with his family. If that sharing is there, all parties can make it through a long hospitalization in a much healthier manner.

### The Need for Privacy

All parents seem to feel an enormous need to simply have time alone with their child to begin building a unique relationship—to do the "silly" things that they may not feel comfortable doing in front of a room of nurses, physicians, and strangers. Always being in full view of a crowd and "on stage" prohibits many from ever being able to do anything other than hold their baby and whatever else the nurse may ask them to do. This again raises the issue of control and permission. Privacy seems to be mentioned as a limiting factor more often by fathers than by mothers.

The family, including siblings, needs private space at least occasionally to have their own family group together. The positive impact of sibling visits to the NICU has been studied and includes better understanding of the parents' love and concern for the baby in the hospital and concrete evidence of the sibling's existence. In some cases, regressive behavior that was observed in the sibling at home before the hospital visit was reversed.[5] It is important, however, to institute a comprehensive policy to screen for infection or recent exposure to communicable diseases (like chicken pox) to ensure safety for the already compromised hospitalized infant.

### The Need for Continuity and Consistency from All Those Involved in the Infant's Care

Consistency seems best accomplished by having a primary team which may include physicians, nurses, social workers, dieticians, and respiratory, occupational, and physical therapists for each chronic child. Primary nursing, for example, without consistency in the medical management cannot overcome the constant monthly changes the parents feel that they and the child go through. If trust can be developed in a core group of staff, the needs of the family, the infant, and the staff can be handled better. Monthly physician rotations are particularly stressful for families, as they must adjust to another attending physician's ethics and treatment plans. The overall medical plan can best be coordinated by an identified primary physician. In some settings, a nurse practitioner oversees the care of infants with chronic hospitalizations and is able to coordinate and communicate the medical plan to the parents. However, if either arrangement is not feasible in a particular setting, a meeting between the physician going off service with the oncoming physician and the parents can clarify goals and previous plans.[2]

### The Need for an Agreed Upon Plan for the Chronic Child Toward Which All Efforts Are Directed

This plan would be arrived at by primary team members, taking into account both the child's medical and developmental needs and the family's needs. Whenever possible, the family should be able to participate in the evolution of this plan. This may lessen some of the usual confusion about how the child is doing, clarify his strengths and weaknesses, and communicate definite milestones that need to be achieved. A plan becomes especially important as the issues of discharge arise, for the parents must know at what level of stability the child must be before discharge is possible.

### The Need for Emotional Support

The family must be supported from the very beginning in handling the emotions that a premature birth and chronic illness produce. A person not directly involved in patient care, usually a social worker or clinical nurse specialist, is generally in the best position to serve the family in this manner. The family must be helped through the initial shock and throughout the transition of trying to learn how to feel like a parent to such a special child and under such unusual conditions. So many factors continue their stress—tiredness, frustration, fear, concern about bills, feeling incompetent to handle such responsibility, anger, and on and on. There must be nonjudgmental support for the family, no matter where they are in the process of working through their feelings.

A social worker who has developed a relationship of trust and understanding with the family can relay their needs and frustrations to the staff. The family may never directly express such needs for fear of "asking too much." This liaison with an "outsider" can also give parents the permission to "let down" with someone when they need to express some of their feelings and frustrations. Even in supportive relationships, there are often issues one partner does not feel are acceptable to talk about with the other partner. A third party can sometimes help everyone involved—including the medical staff—get through a long ordeal a little better.

Maintaining the alliance between staff and family may allow the needs of the infant, family, and staff to be met; a disruption can make the already difficult situation of chronic illness and long hospitalization even worse.[2]

### The Need to Learn the Infant's Care Needs as Soon as Feasible and to Participate in the Care as Much as Possible

A process of "normalization" (mentioned in the case study of Rachel's family) is being incorporated into some NICUs to deal with the consequences to the infant of an intensive care environment and long hospitalization.[6] The three primary principles of this process are (1) recognition of each infant's unique temperament and stage of development, (2) observation of the infant's behavior to determine type and timing of intervention, and (3) the necessity of parent participation. This process facilitates normal survival of baby, staff, and parent.

Areas set aside just for chronic patients can offer privacy for the family as well as a more normal setting for the growing infant. The existence of such areas can encourage flexibility in meeting the infant's developmental needs and simulate a more homelike setting for the family.[7]

Another valuable resource, one used in my own nursery, is having trained volunteers and foster grandmothers who are available to rock, love, and provide more "normal" time for these chronic children. These persons not only benefit the child, but help the parents feel that their child is being held and loved when they are not able to be there.

The NICU staff often helps parents whose infants die to "build memories." It is important to do the same for the parents of chronic infants. They all live with the fear somewhere in their mind that their child may never come home—and this is usually a real possibility. By allowing participation in care, involving siblings and grandparents, keeping diaries, taking photographs, and saving hair and the like, the staff can help the family feel the baby is real—someone who can be known to people outside the walls of the intensive care nursery.

Dealing with chronically ill infants obligates us to do better in dealing with their parents. We must begin to change the often sterile and rule-oriented mode of hospitals to meet the multifaceted needs of these infants and their families. In doing so, we may discover that we better meet the needs of and reduce the stress for the staff. We are dealing with a new kind of patient in the child with chronic lung disease. New and creative solutions are required to meet their needs, their family's needs, and the staff's needs.

## The Abandoned Infant

In both of the case studies, the family was involved from the onset with the care of their child and was able to ask and/or demand participation and inclusion. This is certainly not always the case, particularly in the larger NICUs located in urban areas, where a greater variety of social problems exists. The increase in drug abuse, alcoholism, unintended/unwanted pregnancies, poor prenatal care, and teen pregnancies add to the risk factors that may make a mother or family even more likely not to be involved with the baby—particularly if the infant's problems persist and demand more than a caregiver feels capable of giving.

Rather than getting "lost" at some point during the hospitalization, some families seem never to really be involved with their infant. Their story is often the same: an undesired pregnancy confirmed too late for other options, no prenatal care; a history of drug, alcohol, or tobacco use or mental illness; and/or a complex and multiproblem social system. To these risk factors, we must now add that of the growing number of AIDS and HIV positive mothers and babies. This multiproblem population seems to be producing a significant number of the very small babies who become the chronic residents of the neonatal units. Working with multiproblem families is challenging and can be emotionally depleting for the staff. Some of the difficulties encountered by various health professionals include personal anger and frustration as well as a multitude of institutional and community constraints.[8] If attempts to engage the parents in some type of meaningful relationship with their infant are unsuccessful, what are the consequences? Who then provides for the infant's nurturing while he remains in the hospital? What systems are in place to provide for his needs when he is ready for discharge?

In most cases, the hospital staff, by necessity, must provide the nurturing these infants need. The infants seem to become "claimed" fairly quickly, particularly as the maternal/family history becomes known by staff. A nurse will "adopt" one as her special baby, filling in for the absent family. This commitment can also be the source of pain and loss for the staff member. Consider the case of Gail, a 560 gram, 27 week female with moderate respiratory distress syndrome at birth who went on to develop BPD. Her mother was 22 years old, had four other children, and had received no care during her pregnancy. While the mother was in the hospital, she visited Gail infrequently despite expressing "concern" and "love" for the baby. After the mother's discharge from the hospital, she was not able to be located by phone or by mail—nor did she reappear during the child's six months of hospitalization.

This child had no guardian, no visitors, and no advocate other than the hospital staff, who, by necessity, became her "family." How does the staff deal with their own feelings of anger at this family, meet the infant's needs, and arrange for some suitable placement for this infant in whom they have invested so much of themselves?

In order to meet the emotional/nurturing needs of such infants, NICU staffs must often be creative in their approaches. My own nursery at Grady Hospital in Atlanta, Georgia, began a volunteer program in our NICU seven years ago with the intent of providing more nurturing and normal experiences for our infants—particularly those with prolonged hospital stays, those whose parents are in a distant city or do not visit regularly, and those who are a social/medical placement problem. Volunteers are assigned infants who can benefit from being held, talked to, rubbed, fed, or just having time spent with them. The social worker orients, assigns, and supervises the volunteers and is familiar with the infants and their social and medical problems. The physical therapist often requests that the volunteers do certain activities with the infants and updates these as the infant's age and needs change. The volunteers continue to work with the infant until he is ready for discharge.

This program not only has added to the overall development of infants with long hospital stays, but it has been essential in meeting the complex needs of those infants who are abandoned or have placement problems. Beyond this, the volunteers have been able to give a boost to the staff and help offset some of their feelings of not meeting these infants' emotional needs.

Another program in many nurseries is the foster grandparent program, which functions in much the same way as the volunteer program just described. In my own nursery, the grandmothers provide nurturing for two infants four hours daily and are generally assigned to those infants who need daily, consistent touch and love.

The dilemma of the placement problem ends up being a social issue. Even though the social worker and/or staff can usually identify a problem situation very early on, the systems that exist to look out for infants and children generally fall short of addressing their needs. The gaps widen even further when the child involved is considered a medically high-risk child as well as a socially high-risk infant. The child protective service agencies are often reluctant to get involved, in large part because they know they have few resources (foster homes or alternative placements) that can meet the child's medical needs. Because few alternatives exist, the child may be sent to his natural parents' home or to a relative although *all* those involved (staff, social workers, community agencies) realize that this is probably not in the best interest of a child in whom they have invested so much both emotionally and financially.

If children with special care needs are removed from their natural family or are placed for adoption, their fate may then be to become one of the many "boarder babies" who now live in hospitals across the country because there are no places available to meet their needs. They may remain in institutions for indefinitely prolonged periods of time. Despite the best efforts of staff, the total needs of these children cannot be met in such a setting, and they place tremendous demands on an already inadequate nursing staff.

What is the answer to this growing dilemma? There must be creative thinking about developing alternative placement and permanent homes for these children. Aggressive recruitment of foster homes, encouragement of new types of homes that can meet the medical and emotional needs of the chronic, medically needy, HIV positive, and/or other hard-to-place infants must begin now because the children exist now. This problem calls for the most imaginative thinking by new coalitions of concerned citizens, organizations, and health professionals. We owe no less to these children, who deserve a chance to have what all are entitled to have: security, safety, and nurturing in an environment that fosters their physical and emotional development.

## References


1. Miller LG: Toward a greater understanding of the parents of the mentally retarded child, Journal of Pediatrics 73, 1968, pp. 699–705.
2. Zeanah C, and Jones J: Maintaining the parent-staff alliance in an intensive care nursery, Psychosomatics 23(12), December 1982, pp. 1238–1251.
3. Marino B: When nurses compete with parents, Journal of the Association for Care of Children in Hospitals 8(4), Spring 1980, pp. 94–98.
4. Harrison H: The Premature Baby Book, New York, 1983, St. Martin's Press.
5. Maloney M, et al.: A prospective, controlled study of scheduled sibling visits to a newborn intensive care unit, Journal of the American Academy of Child Psychiatry 22(6), 1983, pp. 565–570.
6. Rushton CH: Promoting normal growth and development in the hospital environment, Neonatal Network 4(6), June 1986, pp. 21–30.
7. Kavalhuna R, and Malhight M: Meeting the needs of the extended care NICU patient, Neonatal Network 2(4), February 1984, pp. 19–25.
8. Fields B: Toward a tenacity of commitment: Understanding and modifying institutional practices and individual responses that impede work with multiproblem families, Zero to Three, June 1987, pp. 9–12.

## Bibliography


- Glassanos M: Infants who are oxygen dependent—sending them home, American Journal of Maternal Child Nursing 5, January/February 1980, pp. 42–45.
- Hall-Johnson S: High Risk Parenting: Nursing Assessment and Strategies for the Family at Risk, Philadelphia, 1979, J. B. Lippincott.
- Scherf R: Total patient care of the newborn infant who develops bronchopulmonary dysplasia, Neonatal Network 3(4), February 1985, pp. 28–37.

CHAPTER 8

# The Long Road Home—Suggested Pathways for Hospital Discharge of Infants with Chronic Respiratory Compromise

*Linda Corcoran, RN*
*Children's Hospital of Philadelphia*
*Philadelphia, Pennsylvania*

Shaneeka lies supine, using her left fist to bat randomly at a mobile strung across her crib top. Her lower extremities are hypotonic, her right arm splayed to the side, hampered by scapular retraction. She is alert but smiles only when prompted with a familiar smiling face eight inches midline in front of her own. Around her neck is a snug foam collar to support her tracheostomy tube. A portable cassette player waxes melodic nursery rhymes (which she recognizes) seemingly in time to the ventilator at her bedside (or is it the ventilator rate she knows so well?). Tape and a silastic nasogastric tube cover part of her right cheek; EKG wires wind their way out between the snaps of her sleeper; the infrared sensor on her right index finger continuously monitors her pulse oximetry. She is an intensive care "resident" and former 25 week premature infant, currently 8 months corrected age. She has bronchopulmonary dysplasia (BPD), feeding intolerance, hypotonia, and developmental delay. Her mother, who sits serenely at her infant's bedside, queries nurses, "When can she go home?"

The current climate surrounding hospital reimbursement has led America's health care system to examine its philosophies and practices of inpatient care.

**TABLE 1 ■ Considerations Central to Discharge Candidacy of an Infant with BPD**

1. **Medical Stability**
   - Prognosis
   - Care needs
   - Stability
2. **Family's Capability**
   - Motivated/bonded to infant
   - Resources
     - Stable family/caretaking group
     - Housing situation: space, utilities, flexibility
     - Community facilities and agencies
     - Available to handle infant needs
   - Ability to learn infant care
   - Ability to independently provide infant care
3. **Availability of Funds**
   - Supplemental Security Income/Dependent Persons Welfare Assistance
   - Third-party payer support/allowances (insurance coverage)

Few issues are as morally and physiologically complex as long-term care of the neonate affected by chronic pulmonary disease and its sequelae. Our nursery reports that the cost per month for a single ventilator-dependent infant housed in an intensive care area is in excess of $60,000. In contrast, home care costs based on equipment needs and projected eight hours of nursing care per day are $9,200.[1-3] More dramatic than the financial figures is the pervasive psychological damage chronic hospitalization has on a growing infant and family.[4] In many tertiary care facilities, these problematic cases are an ongoing struggle, and certainly each infant presents a unique puzzle to unravel. The central issues are the infant's health status and integration into the family. The acuity of the patient's course and parents' ability to cope with the infant's long hospital course and uncertain outcome frequently work against these objectives.[4,5] Ultimately, the goal is to stabilize the infant's disease process and send a well baby home. For many high-risk neonates with extreme prematurity, meconium aspiration, birth asphyxia, multiple congenital anomalies, or cardiac defects, this is frequently not possible. The infant's disease process reaches a plateau from which there is no immediate or steady state resolution. The infant requires oxygen and perhaps long-term ventilation; nutritional problems arise; apnea of obstructive or central neurological origin becomes an issue, and consequently, all parameters require monitoring. These conditions are diagnosed and controlled in the hospital environment. The family who knows and loves this child is faced with the financial burden of hospitalization, the transportation costs, and the strain on coexisting relationships (other children, extended family, employment responsibilities).[4] They desire to incorporate the infant into their own world—even at the cost of disrupting all their previous realities.

This chapter presents an overview of the discharge process, from patient identification through the complexities of a multidisciplinary model and culminates in the family's ability to take charge of the care of their own child in the home. Discharge planning time is necessarily increased as the complexity of the patient's needs increases. The scope of the following process is designed to accommodate families with children who have chronic lung disease and may require artificial airways, assisted ventilation or oxygen, special feeding regimens (gastrostomy, nasogastric), weekly developmental therapies, and sophisticated monitoring in the home setting.

Children with minimal bronchopulmonary dysplasia, whose home needs are satisfied with supplemental nasal cannula oxygen, usually require less time and fewer services to prepare for discharge. However, even families of children with mild to moderate BPD will require careful discharge planning and ongoing guidance regarding nutritional parameters, because this group of infants has an increased risk of poor weight gain and failure to thrive syndrome. These parents must be able to understand and respond appropriately to their child during respiratory infections or other stressful situations and to follow through on any other special care required.[2,3] (see Appendix D)

## Planning for Discharge

Families frequently express a desire to take their infant home. Ultimately, it becomes the health care team's responsibility to ferret out exactly "who" they wish to take home. The concept of the additional care required for an infant with physiologic and equipment needs is not easily grasped by parents who still have hope for resolution of their baby's illness prior to discharge. Parental denial is often apparent first to the nurses who routinely care for these infants. These nurses are in a position to comprehend the discrepancies between what parents see and are told about their infant's medical problems and what they actually understand. Once the question of discharge is raised in informal communication between the family and nurses, actual discharge planning can begin. It is enlightening to observe how consideration of the concrete reality of taking the baby home can open the door of understanding for most families.

The discharge process is complex and multidisciplinary. Prior to any discussion or large-scale planning, three areas must be explored: (1) the infant's medical stability, (2) the family's willingness and capability to assume infant care in their home, and (3) the availability of funds (Table 1).

**TABLE 2 ■ Resource Network for Discharge Process**

| Hospital Multidisciplinary Team | Home Care Resources |
|---|---|
| Nursing staff | VNA/nursing agency |
| Attending MD | Private duty nurses |
| Social workers | Local MD |
| Respiratory therapists | Dependent persons welfare agency/insurance company |
| Infant development services | Equipment company |
| Occupational, physical, and speech therapists | Community rehabilitation programs |
| Equipment safety personnel | Home therapists |
| | Extended family |
| | Community agencies (rescue squad, local emergency room, utilities) |

Nursing staff may discover that the forum of medical rounds or interdisciplinary team rounds is appropriate for initial discussion of these issues.[6] Social workers or in-house personnel responsible for ongoing communication with third-party payers (insurance companies) and/or state and federal agencies should be involved from the moment home care planning begins. It is painful to note that although our concern is patient stability and preparing the parents to take charge of their infant's care, discharge may be temporarily or permanently blocked by lack of funding for care at home.

## A Multidisciplinary Process

The disciplines involved in the discharge process (Table 2) need to focus on the patient and the family. Nursing professionals must take the lead in defining role responsibilities. Although many nurses are required to take part in the physical care of the infant, one should be designated to assume the leadership role in organizing the discharge process. This primary nurse should also have a management supervisor (head nurse, clinical nurse specialist, or hospital nursing discharge coordinator) who will support the efforts of the entire nursery staff and meet routinely with them to solve problems and give guidance and suggestions for meeting projected goals.

The primary nurse should, upon agreement with physicians and social workers, set up a small group meeting with the parents, attending physician, social worker, and herself in attendance. This meeting should set the tone for the entire discharge process by establishing an agreement or contract between the family and hospital personnel, as well as generally outline what is necessary for patient discharge. Although this meeting may be intimidating for the parents, it is often helpful in facilitating a realistic discharge plan: The family can see how complex this undertaking is and how serious their level of commitment needs to be.

Following this family meeting, the nurse, physician, and social worker should discuss their impressions of family reaction and negotiate the next steps in the process: (1) documentation/written goals for family preparation and education, (2) correspondence and agreements with home care funding and provider agencies, and (3) medical consultations and summaries necessary for the plan of home care. Although these responsibilities routinely fall to nurse, social worker, and physician, respectively, they should be officially assigned as soon as possible.

### Parent Education

The primary nurse should design an educational plan for the parents based on the patient's hospital care plan. Parents should be expected to handle well baby care first and then add additional responsibilities. The infant's regular nurses should have an opportunity to participate in changing or contributing to the teaching plan before it is presented to the parents. This presents a single plan of information, thus preventing the conflicting messages that can be generated as each staff member has contact with the family. The plan should include each activity the home caretakers will need to carry out: bathing, exercise, medication administration, nasogastric feedings, equipment operation (oxygen, nasal cannula, tracheostomy care, ventilator, suction machine, monitor), and CPR training. The teaching plan is probably best designed as a checklist with spaces for demonstrations and return demonstrations, as well as written guidelines specifying how each component should be carried out. (see Appendix D)

Once the nursing team has agreed on the written plan, the primary nurse should meet with the family and social worker to review and amend it. This final plan should present a clear picture of the care required and a reasonable timetable for meeting the projected discharge date (Table 3).[7,8]

### Home Funding

Communication with federal, state, and local dependent persons agencies (such as State Welfare/Supplemental Security Income agencies) or private insurance companies should begin as soon as the discharge plan is initiated.[8] Usually this application is initiated by the parent under the supervision of the social worker or discharge coordinator. The written format necessarily includes claimant forms from the funding agency. Additional content should be developed by physicians, the respiratory therapist, and nurses to include

**TABLE 3 ■ Timetable for Discharge of an Infant with BPD**

| | WEEK 1 | WEEK 2 | WEEK 3 | WEEK 4 | WEEK 5 | WEEK 6 |
|---|---|---|---|---|---|---|
| ***Family*** | Expresses desire to care for infant in home environment | Plan home care with assistance of health care team<br><br>Begin active role in well baby care | Verbalize understanding of infant's physiologic issues<br><br>Begin participation in trach/equipment care<br><br>Home modifications<br>1. electrical<br>2. intercom<br>3. telephone | PARENT MEETING<br>Multidisciplinary planning session to assist parents in focusing on their needs and to complete master plan for patient's projected discharge<br>Training and return demonstrations | Training and return demonstrations<br><br>CPR/monitor classes | Responsible for all infant care for 24 hours<br><br>All equipment to home |
| ***Infant development team*** | | Initial evaluation of patient | Meet with family, RN, MD to discuss developmental needs, physiologic parameters of infant's course | | Meet with home therapists | |
| ***Respiratory therapy*** | | Provide recommendations and equipment list for patients including ventilation/respiratory supports necessary at home | Establish plan to train parents in equipment maintenance/troubleshooting | PARENT MEETING<br>Teaching for equipment company, family, home nursing services | Teaching for family, home nursing services | |
| ***Physician*** | Identify patient as candidate [illegible] | Complete and send patient [illegible] | Continue evaluation of patient [illegible] | PARENT MEETING<br>Continue ongoing [illegible] | Confirm services to be provided local medical [illegible] | Send discharge medical summary to local [illegible] |

| | | | | | | |
|---|---|---|---|---|---|---|
| | for additional services (infant development team, OT, PT, speech therapy, nutrition, child life)<br>Contract with parent(s) for viability of home care | insurance company<br>Complete immunization record | ress; provide interim guidance to family regarding home care | cation with family | doctor: follow-up responsibilities | medical doctor |
| ***Nursing*** | Develop short- and long-range goals with parents/caretakers for their assumption of care | Provide additional information for insurance coverage/equipment lists; plan patient home needs | Train parents/caretakers<br>Establish home plan with parents to include additional ordered/child services | PARENT MEETING<br>Train home nursing service<br>Visit home | Train home nursing service | Provide continuing support to family |
| ***Social services*** | Provide parents with community contacts for required future services<br>Institute meetings with parents and insurance company immediately | Assist family in choosing<br>• equipment company<br>• home nursing agency<br>• developmental services<br>• emergency services<br>–ambulance<br>–local ER<br>–utility companies<br>–home pediatrician | Act as resource to family in dealing with insurance company and suppliers | PARENT MEETING<br>Visit home for assessment | Provide continuing support to family | |

patient diagnosis, prognosis, itemized listings of disposable and durable supplies (including equipment, amounts specifically needed, and cost per item), services and agencies required for home care, and projected cost per month of home care in comparison to hospital expenses. In order to expedite the process for the paying organizations, all documentation reviewed and signed by the physician of record should be delivered to the funding agency as soon as the information is completed (not more than one week after the family has initiated discharge planning).

### Consults

In preparation for services in the home, the medical staff needs to compile an overview of the patient's existing problems and deficits; subspecialties should be consulted for updated or new information concerning known patient problems. Frequently these will include ophthalmology, audiology, gastrointestinal/nutrition services, developmental specialties, occupational and physical therapy, speech, educational services, and otolaryngology. All consultations should be undertaken during the first week of planning to determine final projections of services the physician will need to order for home care.

## Parental Decisions

While all this paperwork is being prepared by the hospital staff, the primary focus should continue to be on further establishing the infant-parent relationship and the parent's ability to comprehend the infant's basic pathophysiology in order to translate these problems to caregiving. Two weeks into the educational process, the parents should be able to comprehend what is expected of them and be able to verbalize their role. One nurse, physician, and social worker should meet with the parents to discuss anxieties, frustrations, and fears that the family may be experiencing. Many families may be feeling pressured or out of control by this point. Above all, they need assurance that the infant's needs and their own are central to the process and that they can control the tempo of planning and eventual discharge. Parents must be encouraged to communicate their concerns about the discharge plan and know they can stop the process at any time. These types of infants and families do not respond well to absolute deadlines established by the health care team, and it is better to delay discharge than to send the infant home to an unprepared family. It is critical to reinforce the issue of transfer of responsibility from hospital staff to parents at this time and throughout the remainder of the infant's hospitalization.

### Home Nursing Care

Hospital staff should find out how much assistance the family will need in caring for the infant at home.[8-10] The complexity of care will dictate whether the family needs in-home nursing care or a visiting nurse referral. If the parent's decision is to employ nurses in the home, the social worker or the discharge coordinator may suggest several agencies that are available in the family's geographical area. An alternative is to have the family privately advertise and recruit nurses independently. The family, as the employer, must make the final hiring decisions concerning nurses who work in their home. Although hospital personnel should offer them guidance through the interview and selection process, the family needs to direct the interviewing and screening of applicants.

Two critical issues here will be the funding available to the family and the nursing services available in their community. For example, an infant who requires assisted ventilation via tracheostomy also needs suctioning at least every 3–4 hours. In the very best scenario—an intact family with two trained parents—private nursing services must be employed for at least 8 hours per day. (Our experience with such situations has been that nursing personnel in the home 24 hours a day at least initially is a requirement for family integrity and emotional stability.) Visiting nurse assistance is usually appropriate when the infant's care is limited to supplemental oxygen therapy and/or special feeding needs. These recommendations may become a problem when funding is limited to a specific state or county approved nursing agency (as opposed to a privately financed agency) that cannot provide the technically prepared nurses for home care.

### Medical Equipment

Parents should be advised of options that are available to them in their community. Hospital respiratory therapists are involved in selecting the best possible equipment for home support. Selection of an equipment company should be based on the vendor's ability to: (1) deliver all equipment to the home, (2) have available registered respiratory therapists on a 24-hour emergency service basis, and (3) work with the family to correct equipment failures and negotiate payment issues.[10] The parents should meet with representatives of the prospective company and present the equipment lists to their funding agencies. Although hospital staff may have a past working relationship with a particular company, the family should make the final choice of vendor. However, insurance companies may also determine the vendor, as many have established "contracts" in order to reduce costs. It is important to determine in such cases that the insurance company's selected vendor has suitable equipment and services, and that they have experience dealing with pediatric patients.

### Community Services

Parents must identify a number of resources close to their home for emergency situations, including a pediatrician, hospital emergency room, ambulance company/fire rescue squad, utility companies (electric, heat, telephone), and child services (developmental program, and occupational, physical, and speech therapists). These services may require documentation from the attending physician to verify the infant's current disposition and projected time until resolution of illness.

When all agencies have been contracted by the parents, a family meeting should be scheduled, at least one month prior to the infant's projected discharge date. This forum should be attended by representatives of all hospital disciplines involved in the patient's care along with services that will be taking part in the home care. Although the meeting is usually mediated by the discharge coordinator, the parents/caretakers should be encouraged to participate freely in these proceedings.

## Home Preparation

Shortly after the planning forum, one or two members of the hospital team should meet with the parents in their home. This visit should be used as an opportunity for the parents to explain how they have prepared or altered their living space to accommodate their infant. If at all possible, a small room or area on the first floor should be designated as the infant's space. This may afford other family members privacy and minimize interference by nurses, therapists, and other personnel. Every piece of equipment necessary for care should be planned for; electrical amperage upgrades may be necessary to support equipment function. The family and equipment company should reach an agreement about placement of primary monitors, oxygen, ventilator, and suction machines, and arrangements should be made for backup equipment storage.

### Parent Education

By week four of discharge planning, three individuals should be accomplished in well baby care and the basic techniques of special care the infant requires. These three persons may be a single parent and his or her designates (grandparents, neighbors, other family members) but must be the three individuals who will be coordinating infant care in the home. The time line from week four until discharge is entirely dependent on how comfortable these individuals feel and how well they are progressing toward independence in caregiving. In addition to routine care, emergency situations must be carefully reviewed. CPR teaching and classes in troubleshooting monitors and any other equipment necessary for home care (ventilator, resuscitator bag, continuous feeding pump) are an essential component of parent training.

Lastly, the parents should assume total responsibility for infant care. This may be accomplished in the hospital with the use of home equipment. The parents should be responsible for all infant care between 8 to 24 hours. An alternative is an 8-hour home pass, during which the parents care for their child at home under the supervision of an intensive care nurse. This "dress rehearsal" allows the parents to assume responsibility for their infant with hospital staff present to come to their aid should they become uncertain of an emergency procedure.

### Home Services Education

Home care nursing personnel and home infant developmental therapists should meet the family prior to discharge. If home nursing staff has had prior experience with another patient with similar problems, an 8-hour training period that includes time for hands-on care of the infant is usually sufficient. This time frame should allow hospital staff to review patient history and home care plans with the home nurses. In most instances, this predischarge use of home nursing time will be attributed to orientation of staff by the funding agency. Most importantly, all home nurses and at least one fire rescue squad member should have hospital-based basic life-support training adapted to the infant's individual needs.

## Medical Readiness for Discharge

Although all else may be prepared to transfer a chronically ill infant to his home, the child cannot be discharged until he establishes and maintains specific baseline physiologic criteria (Table 4).

Once parameters are at acceptable levels, the hospital attending physician should negotiate with the appointed local pediatrician to establish a plan for noninvasive monitoring (to be performed as scheduled by the home respiratory therapists), as well as a plan for direction and management of postdischarge oxygen weaning, medication changes, and nutritional supervision. A written discharge summary should be completed by the hospital physician, with copies sent to the home pediatrician, community emergency room, and parents.

**TABLE 4 ▪ Baseline Physiologic Criteria Indicating Patient's Medical Readiness for Discharge**

1. **Airway Stability:**
   Arterial $PaO_2$, $PCO_2$ measurements within reasonable physiologic limits for disease state
   Pulse oximetry ≥ 90% during all activity levels or plan to change therapy to support changes
   End tidal $CO_2$ (≤ 60)
   Pulmonary function testing (if available) at individual baseline for all activities
   - patent airway
   - resistance
   - compliance
   - work of breathing

   Thermistor/pneumocardiogram interpreted for obstructive or central apnea and $O_2$ desaturation during all activities
2. **Medications:** therapeutic levels on adjusted doses of diuretics, bronchodilators, anti-convulsants
3. **Nutrition:** has achieved appropriate rate of growth for gestational age; adequate caloric intake to support individual metabolic rate and growth curve
4. **Thermoregulation:** has established baseline for temperature control

## Conclusion

The sequence suggested in this discussion is based on actual clinical observations made in 31 individual patient/family situations in our intensive care setting. Although each infant's situation determines the resources necessary for completing home care planning, the following factors have been present in the successful discharge of the infants in our nursery:

1. The infant is medically stable, and the family has completed all discharge training.
2. The family has the desire and the ability to care for their infant and his medical needs at home.
3. The hospital team undertakes a collaborative effort that includes the disciplines of nursing, social services, medicine, respiratory therapy, and infant development.
4. The community where the family/infant resides has available the resources that have been identified as necessary for the infant's home care requirements.
5. Equipment and funding for home care meet approved standards for infant safety and care quality as outlined by the discharge team.

The discharge process for an infant with long-term respiratory care needs is arduous and complex. The effort required by all participants is apparent. Yet the benefits gained by integrating the BPD infant into his family and community are great and worth the time and effort. Therefore, health professionals must rise to the challenge of orchestrating a safe discharge for their patients with chronic lung disease.

## References


1. Personal conversation with Elissa Kopf, ACSW, Social Services, Children's Hospital of Philadelphia.
2. Corcoran L, Spitzer AR, and Fox WW: Early discharge for neonates requiring continuing respiratory support, Pediatric Research 19, 1985, p. 402A.
3. McCormick MC, Berbaum J, and Eisenberg J: Observations on the post discharge costs of caring for the VLBW infant, Pediatric Research 23, 1988, p. 452A.
4. Schraeder BD: A creative approach to caring for the ventilator dependent child, The American Journal of Maternal-Child Nursing 4(3), 1979, pp. 165–170.
5. Burr B, et al.: Home care of children on respirators (Massachusetts Department of Public Health), New England Journal of Medicine 309(21), 1983, pp. 1319–1323.
6. Steele NF, and Harrison B: Technology-assisted children: Assessing discharge preparation, Journal of Pediatric Nursing 1(3), 1986, pp. 150–158.
7. Ad hoc task force on home care of chronically ill infants and children: Guidelines for home care of infants, children, and adolescents with chronic disease, Pediatrics 74(3), 1984, pp. 434–436.
8. Schreiner MS, Donar ME, and Kettrick RG: Pediatric home mechanical ventilation, Pediatric Clinics of North America 34(1), 1987, pp. 47–60.
9. Thilo EH, et al.: Home oxygen therapy in the newborn—costs and parental acceptance, American Journal of Diseases of Children 141(7), 1987, pp. 766–788.
10. Hartsell MD, and Ward JH: Selecting equipment vendors for children on home care, The American Journal of Maternal-Child Nursing 10(1), 1985, pp. 26–28.


## Bibliography


- Abman S, Accurso F, and Koops B: Experience with home oxygen in the management of infants with bronchopulmonary dysplasia, Clinical Pediatrics 23(9), September 1984, pp. 471–476.
- Glassanos M: Infants who are oxygen dependent—sending them home, Maternal/Child Nursing 5, January/February 1980, pp. 42–45.
- Kloor T, and Carbajal D: Infant oxygen administration by modified nasal cannula, Clinical Pediatrics 23(9), September 1984, pp. 477–479.
- Koops B, Abman S, and Accurso F: Outpatient management and follow-up of bronchopulmonary dysplasia, Clinics in Perinatology 11(1), February 1984, pp. 101–122.
- Jackson D: Nursing care plan: Home management of children with BPD, Pediatric Nursing 12(5), September/October 1986, pp. 342–348.
- Johns N, and Harvey C: Home care of babies with BPD: A workbook for parents, available through the Philadelphia Parenting Associates, 229 W. Upsal St., Philadelphia, Pennsylvania 19119, (215) 438-7234.

## CHAPTER 9

# Home Ventilation for the Infant with BPD: A Model Program

*Jean Homrighausen Zander, RN, MSN*
*Formerly with Section of Pediatric Pulmonology*
*James Whitcomb Riley Hospital for Children*
*Indianapolis, Indiana*

As technological advances have been made in the care of critically ill infants and children, increasing numbers of these patients are surviving, dependent upon mechanical ventilation, physiological monitoring, or supplemental oxygen. Concurrently, there is a strong movement to minimize health care costs and expedite the transition from hospital to home.[1-3] The Home Ventilator Program at James Whitcomb Riley Hospital for Children in Indianapolis was established to meet the needs of ventilator-dependent children and their families: to provide safe home care, to promote normal growth and development and family dynamics, and to minimize the cost of high-tech care. This chapter presents the elements of discharge planning and the essentials of home care for the ventilator-dependent child as practiced by the Riley program.

### Candidates

The prime indication for the use of home mechanical ventilation is chronic alveolar hypoventilation resulting in respiratory failure with hypoxemia and hypercapnea. Chronic alveolar hypoventilation may occur in the child with airway or parenchymal disease such as bronchopulmonary dysplasia (BPD) or

**FIGURE 1 ■ Etiologies of Chronic Alveolar Hypoventilation**

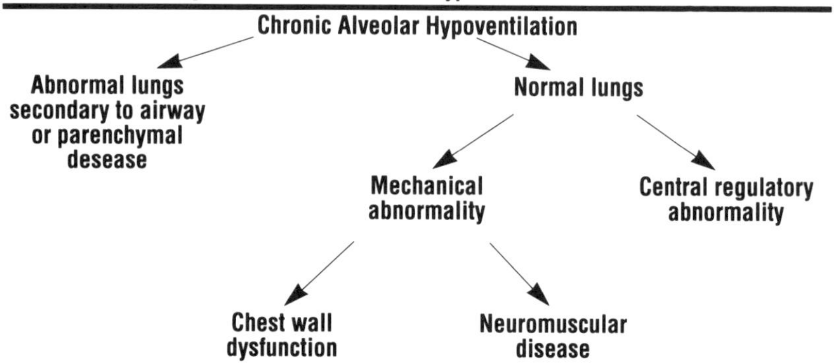


in a child with normal lungs (Figure 1). In the latter instance, a central regulatory abnormality (such as a failure of respiratory drive) or a mechanical dysfunction (such as a chest wall deformity or neuromuscular disease) is the etiology of hypoventilation.[4]

Table 1 presents the diagnostic classification for the 41 patients who have been cared for in the Riley program. Twenty of these children (48.7 percent) have a neuromuscular disease such as muscular dystrophy and Werdnig-Hoffman disease; an additional six children have a neuromuscular disease with concomitant kyphoscoliosis designated as a "mixed" chest/neuromuscular abnormality. Five children (12 percent) have a disorder of central regulation; seven (17 percent) have severe BPD. General data on the current home ventilator population and data on patients who have been weaned from mechanical ventilation are listed in Table 2.

Although pediatric home ventilation candidates include a variety of ages and diagnoses, these children have many needs in common. The complex discharge planning process must be preceded by a thorough assessment of the child and family. The child must undergo medical evaluation to verify "true" ventilator dependence: an inability to maintain adequate ventilation in a child who is free of respiratory infection and is well nourished. Prior to discharge, the child's medical status must be stable. Parameters for stability are somewhat subjective and depend upon the judgment of the attending physician, but Goldberg has proposed criteria for medical stability which we have employed in selected instances.[3] (Table 3)

Home assessment begins with a discussion of the family's readiness to take the child home. Parents must be informed of the long-term responsibility and

**TABLE 1 ■ Riley Hospital Home Ventilator Program: Patient Classification by Diagnosis (May 1988)**

| | Airway or Parenchymal Disease | Primary Chest Wall Abnormality | Primary Neuromuscular Disease | Central Regulatory Disorder | Total |
|---|---|---|---|---|---|
| At home, on ventilation | 4 | — | 15 | 1 | 20 |
| At home, weaned from ventilation | 1 | 2 | 1 | — | 4 |
| Transferred care to another center | — | — | 3 | 2 | 5 |
| Died | — | — | 2 | 2 | 4 |
| Referred from other centers | — | — | 4 | — | 4 |
| Discharge from hospital pending | 2 | 1 | 1 | — | 4 |
| Total | 7 | 3 | 26 | 5 | 41 |

risks they are undertaking. The family may be unable or unwilling to assume this commitment; the home may be small or unsafe. However, in Indiana and in many parts of the country, there are few or no extended care facilities equipped to assume care for the ventilator-dependent child with BPD. Thus, we have worked closely with some families to *make* the home suitable for discharge, even if our initial assessment was not encouraging.

Many adults can assume at least partial responsibility for their own care, but infants and young children obviously cannot. Because they are totally dependent upon others, planning for children requires assessing the needs of the entire family. A keystone for success in home ventilator management is adequate support for the family. Based upon the child's home care needs, the family schedule, and the degree of involvement of extended family, arrangements are made for private duty nursing care in the home.

## The Hospital-Based Home Ventilator Program

At Riley Hospital, the multidisciplinary home ventilator team consists of physicians (pulmonary, developmental, and other pediatric subspecialties), pediatric pulmonary clinical nurse specialist, primary staff nurse, social worker, respiratory therapist, physical therapist, occupational therapist, speech therapist, psychologist, and feeding specialist. Outside the hospital, the team members communicate with their primary care counterparts in the child's

**TABLE 2 ■ Riley Hospital Home Ventilator Program**

| Patients Followed (May 1, 1988) | | | | | | | |
|---|---|---|---|---|---|---|---|
| Patient # | Diagnosis | Date Started HMV* | Age HMV* Begun | Ventilator | Hrs on Ventilation | Assistance (per day) | Comments |
| 1 | Neuromuscular disease | 3/77 | 6 years | Iron lung | Night | — | High school student |
| 2 | Neuromuscular disease | 8/10/77 | 13 1/2 years | Iron lung<br>LP6, 1984 | Night<br>24 hours<br>1985 | LPN 8 hours<br>Mon–Fri | Completed high school, unemployed; sibling of patient #5 |
| 3 | Congenital amyotonia | 3/13/78 | 11 1/2 years | Iron lung<br>LP6, 1984 | Night | — | Completed high school, now in college |
| 4 | Congenital Muscular Dystrophy | 7/22/81 | 12 years | Iron lung | Night | — | Home tutor at mother's request, will finish high school in June |
| 5 | Neuromuscular disease | 12/28/83 | 16 1/2 years | LP6 | Night | — | Completed high school, now in vocational school for job training; sibling of patient #2 |
| 6 | Myelomeningocele | 6/1/84 | 15 years | LP4 | Night | — | High school student |
| 7 | Neuromuscular disease | 6/1/84 | 13 years | LP6 | Night<br>24 hours<br>Fall 1986 | — | Single-parent family, mother employed full-time outside home, sister assists with care |
| 8 | Juvenile rheumatoid arthritis with quadriplegia | 6/84 | 11 years | LP6 | 24 hours | Aide/LPN<br>12–16 hours | Home tutor |
| 9 | Werdnig-Hoffman's disease | 2/20/85 | 15 months | LP6 | 24 hours | RN/LPN<br>12 hours | |
| 10 | L-carnitine deficiency | 11/20/85 | 13 months | LP6 | 24 hours | RN/LPN<br>12 hours | Single-parent family, mother employed part-time outside home |
| 11 | Hypodemylinating neuropathy | 12/5/85 | 2 years | LP6 | 24 hours | RN/LPN<br>12 hours | Parents both employed full-time |
| 12 | Werdnig-Hoffman's disease | 6/30/86 | 17 months | LP6 | 24 hours | 12 hours | |

| | | | | | | | |
|---|---|---|---|---|---|---|---|
| 13 | Central Hypoventilation | 8/26/86 | 5 1/2 months | Sechrist IV–100B–F | Night/naps | 12 hours | Active toddler, developmentally normal except speech |
| 14 | Werdnig-Hoffman's disease | 12/23/86 | 16 months | LP6 | 24 hours | 12 hours | |
| 15 | BPD | 3/12/87 | 16 1/2 months | LP6 | 24 hours | 12 hours | Also has complex cyanotic heart disease |
| 16 | Myelomeningocele | 8/24/87 | 12 years | LP6 | Night | — | Attends school |
| 17 | BPD | 10/19/87 | 9 months | LP6 | 24 hours | 12 hours | Both parents employed full-time |
| 18 | Myelomeningocele | 8/28/87 | 19 years | Iron lung LP6, 12/87 | Night | 40 hours/ week | Used iron lung for 3 months with poor results |
| 19 | BPD | 11/12/87 | 3 years | LP6 | Night | 12 hours | Single parent, pregnant |
| 20 | BPD | 2/9/88 | 2 1/2 years | LP6 | 24 hours | 16 hours | Single parent; has 18 month old healthy sibling |
| 21 | Renal Osteodystrophy | 8/3/83 | 20 months | Sechrist | Night | 16 hours | Ventilated 8/83–4/84; successfully weaned in hospital, 6/10/85, after one in-hospital weaning failure |
| 22 | BPD | 5/9/84 | 34 months | Emerson & LP6 | 24 hours Sleep | 24 hours | Weaned at home in fall 1986; ventilated 2 1/2 years, continues to receive 24 hour nursing assistance |
| 23 | Congenital heart disease w/post-op diaphragmatic paralysis | 10/16/85 | 10 1/2 years | Iron lung | Night | — | Weaned at home |
| 24 | Paraplegia secondary to motor vehicle accident | 9/85 | 3 years | LP6 | Night/naps | 12 hours | Weaned at home |

*Home mechanical ventilation

**TABLE 3 ■ Criteria for Medical Stability Among Children with Cardiopulmonary Abnormalities and Those with Healthy Lungs**

| | Children with Cardiopulmonary Abnormalities | Children with Healthy Lungs |
|---|---|---|
| ***Clinical Criteria*** | Positive trend on growth curve with sustained weight gain<br>Stamina for periods of play<br>Freedom from frequent respiratory infection and fever<br>Medically stable with optimal ventilation | Same |
| ***Ventilation Criteria*** | $PaO_2$ >60 torr in $FiO_2 \leq 0.4$ and $PaCO_2 \leq 50$ torr | $PaO_2$ >70 torr in room air and $PaCO_2$ <45 torr |

Adapted from Goldberg AI, et al.: Home care for life supported persons: An approach to program development, Journal of Pediatrics 104(5), 1984, pp. 785–795

home community. We have found that the following factors contribute to program success:

1. The program is coordinated by the tertiary care center and includes primary caregivers.
2. A chronology for implementation and the responsibilities of each team member are specifically delineated (see Appendix E and F).
3. One team member is designated as coordinator or case manager; in our setting, this is the pediatric pulmonary clinical nurse specialist.
4. To promote good communication, all planning and implementation are documented.
5. Prior to discharge, all primary home caregivers (parents, volunteers, and private duty nurses) participate in a hospital-based education program.

Once the initial assessment of the family has been completed, the multidisciplinary team meets under the direction of the clinical nurse specialist to plan for all services and equipment that will be needed in the home (Table 4).

## Equipment Selection

### Ventilator

Ventilation can be provided by negative or positive pressure methods. Research in negative pressure ventilation began in the late nineteenth century.[5] Today's devices operate on the same principle: The chest is enclosed in a tank, the head is exposed, and subatmospheric pressure is applied to the chest to induce inspiration. When pressure within the tank is allowed to return to atmospheric pressure, expiration takes place passively.

An iron lung is easy to operate, inexpensive, and can be hand-operated by crank in the event of electrical failure. In addition, it is sturdy, durable, and

**TABLE 4 ■ Initial Home Planning Meeting**

| *Roster* | *Agenda* |
|---|---|
| Pediatric pulmonologist | 1. Brief review of medical history and discharge planning status |
| Clinical nurse specialist | 2. Determination of need for equipment/supplies<br>Fixed base ventilator<br>Portable ventilator<br>Oxygen<br>Portable suction<br>Electrical suction<br>Wheelchair<br>Hospital bed<br>Automotive restraint system<br>Lift<br>Tracheostomy tubes, suction catheters<br>Gastrostomy tubes, feeding pump, formula<br>Ramps, widened doorways, electrical changes |
| Primary nurse from inpatient unit | |
| Respiratory therapist | |
| Dietitian | |
| Social worker | |
| Occupational therapist | |
| Physical therapist | |
| Speech therapist | 3. Determination of need for services<br>Home nursing care<br>Occupational therapy<br>Physical therapy<br>Speech therapy<br>Specialized transportation (car seat)<br>Education (school vs. home bound)<br>Well-child care<br>Contact electric company/phone company/emergency service |
| Psychologist | |
| Parents (in some cases) | |

needs little maintenance. An artificial airway such as a tracheostomy is not required, and there is no danger of airway disconnection. There is no water reservoir, so there is decreased risk of infection and decreased cleaning time. However, the machine is large and cumbersome and may be difficult to accommodate in the home. Ventilation is by the control mode only, so the patient is unable to vary his own respiratory rate (the I:E ratio is set at 1:1).

Iron lungs are well suited for the patient with neuromuscular disease who requires support only at night, but their use may present problems for other children. For example, a negative pressure device may be unable to generate the high negative pressure needed to ventilate adequately the baby with BPD. The iron lung also produces confinement and physical restriction for an active, developing infant or toddler.

A cuirass or other smaller negative pressure device has several advantages over the traditional iron lung. Care is easier because the body is not totally encased. Many of these devices can provide an "assist" mode rather than just control. However, the cuirass may not supply a full tidal volume to the patient.

Although positive pressure devices are more complex and expensive, they offer finer adjustment of volumes and pressures, essential to the child with

**TABLE 5 ■ Advantages and Disadvantages of Oxygen Sources**

| OXYGEN SYSTEM | ADVANTAGES | DISADVANTAGES |
|---|---|---|
| ***Compressed gas (tanks)*** | Long shelf life<br>Easily available | Heavy<br>Frequent refills<br>High pressure (2,000 PSI)<br>Low volume for size compared with liquid system |
| ***Liquid oxygen*** | Low pressure (20 PSI)<br>Portability<br>Easy home refilling | Evaporation<br>Frostbite during transfilling<br>Technical problems (i.e., ice formation) |
| ***Concentrators and enrichers*** | Simple, easy to use<br>Mobile | Heavy<br>Not portable<br>Need power source |

BPD. Positive pressure ventilators allow the child increased mobility; an internal battery permits the child to be disconnected from an external power source. A major disadvantage of the positive pressure ventilator, however, is the need for a tracheostomy.

### Oxygen Systems

The patient with neuromuscular disease who has normal lungs usually has an oxygen requirement only when he has recurrent atelectasis or infection. In contrast, the infant with BPD may have markedly impaired oxygenation, requiring supplemental oxygen during sleep, during activity, or continuously.

Factors to consider in selecting a home oxygen system include the following:

- Intended usage
- Weight of system
- Ease of refills
- Low flow capacity
- Need for backup
- Home environment
- Local supply and service
- Economics and reimbursement

When deciding between liquid or compressed gas, we consider the type of ventilator to be used and the number of hours of ventilation per day. The advantages and disadvantages of various oxygen systems should be considered in some detail (Table 5).

Other equipment needs may include feeding pumps, wheelchair, ramps, hospital beds, or car seats. We seek to ensure the child's safety while minimiz-

**TABLE 6 ▪ Sample Monthly Baseline Cost For Home Mechanical Ventilation**

| | MONTHLY RENTAL | ONGOING/MONTHLY DISPOSABLE | SINGLE PURCHASE |
|---|---|---|---|
| *Ventilator* | $1,316.00 | $198.00 | $1,097.00 |
| *Alarms and monitors* | $443.00 | $41.82 | $39.40 |
| *Oxygen* | $190.00 | $1,260.00 | $644.00 |
| *Airway care* | $136.65 | $195.43 | $9.90 |
| *Nutritional supplies* | -0- | $200.25 | -0- |
| *Home care services* | -0- | $8,889.01 | -0- |
| *Cleaning and service* | $35.00 | $177.22 | -0- |
| *Specialized equipment* | -0- | -0- | -0- |
| *Riley Hospital home care management* | -0- | $105.00 | $5,307.00 |
| *Total* | $2,120.65 | $11,066.73 | $7,097.30 |

According to this rental proposal, there would be an estimated initial single purchase of $7097.30 and monthly expenditures of $13,187.38.

ing the equipment and supplies introduced into the home. For example, we do not routinely recommend the use of a hospital bed in the home.

## Equipment and Skills

At the conclusion of the initial multidisciplinary planning meeting, the respiratory therapy home care coordinator submits a list of all necessary durable medical equipment to qualified vendors in the area. The vendors return bids, and one is selected based upon quality of service and cost savings.

While bid procurement and vendor selection are taking place, the clinical nurse specialist and social worker meet regularly with the family and primary nurse. A teaching plan is formulated to include all nursing care skills the family must learn before discharge; these skills include gastrostomy tube care, tracheostomy care, medicine administration, and respiratory assessment. The parents and other volunteer caretakers begin to practice these skills, and they provide three return demonstrations of each prior to discharge.

**TABLE 7 ■ Cost Analysis: Home Versus Hospital Projected Home Care Costs**

| | With Rental of Equipment | With Purchase of Equipment |
|---|---|---|
| Year 1 | $165,345.86 | $160,550.21 |
| Daily | $453.00 | $439.86 |
| Year 2 | $158,248.56 | $132,800.76 |
| Daily | $433.56 | $363.84 |
| **Hospital Bill** | | |
| 5-29-87 thru 6-29-87 | $27,716.79 | $894.09 daily |
| 6-29-87 thru 7-29-87 | $25,715.07 | $857.17 daily |
| 7-29-87 thru 8-29-87 | $23,219.13 | $752.23 daily |

## Third-Party Payment

The hospital patient accounts representative provides the clinical nurse specialist with a description of insurance coverage and the name of a contact person within the insurance corporation. The clinical nurse specialist prepares a home care proposal listing all equipment and services needed for home care along with the rental or purchase price (Table 6) and justification for each item. Included in the cost summary is an estimate of the average daily home care cost analyzed in relation to the child's "maintenance care" hospital bill (Table 7). This information is then submitted to the third-party payer to document the cost savings achieved by home care. Early in our program, we found this step to be the most frustrating to family and team alike. Many third-party payers were unprepared to deal with the extensive home care needs of these children. However, as the insurance industry recognizes the financial advantages of home versus hospital care, they are developing individual case management programs and provision for extracontractual consideration.

## Home Nursing Care

No parents can be expected to care for their ventilator-dependent child 24 hours every day, indefinitely, without relief or assistance. Thus, an important facet of the nursing role is to work with the parents in finding caretakers to assist them.

We encourage the family to find volunteers, but we have had very little success with this; few family members or friends want to assume such responsibility. Most families must rely on private duty nursing assistance. Of our 20 current home ventilator patients, 7 families manage home care without private duty nursing, 1 of whom has a child who is ventilated 24 hours every day but is unable to secure assistance because of problems with third-party pay-

**TABLE 8 ▪ Riley Hospital Home Ventilator Program: Home Care Assistance**

| VENTILATOR ASSISTANCE | NUMBER OF PATIENTS | PAID ASSISTANCE (RN OR LPN) |
|---|---|---|
| *Part-time* | 1 | 40 hours per week |
| | 2 | 12 hours per day |
| | 6 | -0- |
| *Full-time* | 1 | 16 hours per day |
| | 8 | 12 hours per day |
| | 1 | 40 hours per week |
| | 1 | -0- |

ment. (Six children and adolescents in this group are on night or "sleep" assistance alone and do not need assistance.) The remaining 13 patients (12 families) receive assistance that ranges from 40 hours each week to 16 hours each day (Table 8). This nursing care offers respite for the parents and may enable them to maintain employment outside the home.

Home care nurses can be secured through an agency or by advertising in the local news media. We have found advantages and disadvantages inherent in both methods. An agency relieves the parents of much administrative responsibility (such as scheduling and payroll), but tends to remove an element of control the parents may wish to retain in their child's care. If an agency is selected, the administrator must be aware of the philosophy of the home ventilator program and the responsibilities the agency nurses are expected to fulfill. Prior to training the nurses, the clinical nurse specialist, primary nurse, and family meet with the agency to convey these expectations.

Many rural areas of Indiana lack home nursing agencies. In these regions, the clinical nurse specialist and social worker help the family secure private duty nurses. Families advertise in the newspaper, in church bulletins, and on the radio. They have also found it advantageous to contact local hospitals and employment offices for names of nurses seeking part-time, flexible employment. The clinical nurse specialist can provide the family with sample "want ads" and employment applications and can role-play employment interviews.

Although many parents may supervise employees in their workplace, few have been in the position of serving as an employer of someone in their own home. We point out to parents the importance of maintaining a professional relationship with nurses and explain the "how to" of such a relationship. For example, we encourage parents to have the nurses fill out applications and be interviewed. We provide the parents with applications and interview guidelines when necessary (see Appendix F). We emphasize that the daily presence of a "stranger" in the home can add stress and awkwardness to the environment and impact the family's lifestyle.

Many families have spent a lengthy time in the hospital, have formed deep friendships with inpatient nurses, and seek this same friendship as a basis for relationships with home care nurses. We have *repeatedly* seen this approach create problems in the home situation; many families find it difficult to confront the care issues of their child when they have established a close friendship with the nursing staff.

## Caretaker Training

When the third-party payer has approved the home care proposal, a discharge date is selected, and the caretaker training schedule is finalized. All caretakers (defined as parents, volunteers, and paid nurses) acquire certification in infant or child CPR prior to the training program. They are taught specific resuscitation for the child with a tracheostomy, relying upon the use of a manual resuscitation bag.

The 40-hour training program is provided by the home ventilator team. The first two 8-hour days consist of classroom instruction in operating the ventilator, oxygen system, suction machines, and other necessary equipment. In addition, physical therapy, occupational therapy, speech therapy, and child psychology/behavioral specialists discuss the specific home program for the child. Parents, nurses, and any volunteers participate together in these sessions. At the conclusion of the classroom instruction, each caretaker performs a return demonstration of the operation and cleaning of all equipment. The caretaker is then considered capable of beginning bedside training in the inpatient unit with the ventilator-dependent child. Each caretaker must care for the child for three 8-hour shifts prior to discharge, demonstrate all specialized nursing care procedures three times, and complete two additional demonstrations on equipment.

Approximately two weeks prior to discharge, the home care vendor meets with the family, clinical nurse specialist, primary nurse, and home nursing agency coordinator to discuss equipment delivery and arrangements in the home. The electrical system has been assessed and provisions made for rewiring if necessary. In addition, the family has arranged readily accessible storage areas and has devised a schedule for equipment cleaning and maintenance.

## Tracheostomy Care

Obviously, the small pediatric trachea requires a smaller tracheostomy tube. These small tubes cannot accommodate an inner cannula, a cuff, or a fenestra-

**TABLE 9 ■ Shiley Tracheostomy Tubes**

| SIZE | OUTER DIAMETER (MM) | INNER DIAMETER (MM) | NEONATAL LENGTH | PEDIATRIC LENGTH |
|---|---|---|---|---|
| 00 | 4.5 | 3.1 | 30 | 39 |
| 0 | 5.0 | 3.4 | 32 | 40 |
| 1 | 5.5 | 3.7 | 34 | 41 |
| 2 | 6.0 | 4.1 | — | 42 |
| 3 | 7.0 | 4.8 | — | 44 |
| 4 | 8.0 | 5.5 | — | 46 |

tion. (A fenestration, available in larger tubes, is a small opening in the dorsum of the tube. When the tube is plugged, it allows passage of air into the upper airway, promoting vocal cord tone and permitting vocalization.)

Many commercially available tracheostomy tubes won't fit the infant or toddler. A tube that will fit through the stoma into the tracheal lumen may be too long, irritating the carina or entering a mainstem bronchus.

Table 9 shows an example of the limited selection of pediatric tracheostomy tubes. The smallest Shiley brand tubes, both neonatal and pediatric sizes, are listed. The problem arises when a child who is using a #1 neonatal tube must move to the next largest size—the #2 pediatric. There is only a small change in outer diameter (0.5 mm) but an 8 mm change in length. Thus, care may be complicated by limited selection. We have worked with design engineers to obtain custom manufacture of a variety of tube lengths; in addition, we have used custom-manufactured cuffed tracheostomy tubes for some ventilator-dependent infants.

The small lumen of the tracheostomy tube may easily be occluded by thick secretions in the infant with BPD. Strict attention must be paid to providing adequate humidification and to suctioning. Skin care may also be a problem. The tracheostomy tube strings may irritate the skin on the short, fat necks of babies and toddlers—in some cases producing open wounds. We have successfully prevented this by applying Stomahesive as a "cushion" on the neck, beneath the ties. Specially made devices such as Dale tracheostomy tube holders may also prevent irritation; however, due to the Velcro attachments on these ties, they are not suitable for active, inquisitive children.

We discharge all infants and toddlers who have a tracheostomy with an apnea/bradycardia monitor. Although the standard impedance monitor will continue to detect the labored respiratory movements taking place against an obstructed airway, the bradycardia monitor will detect a drop in heart rate, alerting the parents. Monitors that detect flow by changes in temperature or carbon dioxide are also available, but they are more expensive, difficult to use,

**TABLE 10 ■ Summary of Home Care Teaching for Parents of Child with Tracheostomy**

***Prior to discharge from the hospital, parents must demonstrate the following skills:***

1. Explain normal anatomy of trachea, and describe relationship between trachea and esophagus.
2. State reason for tracheostomy.
3. Name parts of tracheostomy tube and purpose of each.
4. State importance of humidification, method of delivery, and care of equipment.
5. Demonstrate suctioning techniques using suction catheter, bulb syringe, and portable suction trap. Demonstrate care and cleaning of suction machine.
6. Demonstrate cleaning of inner cannula.
7. Demonstrate instillation of normal saline and indications for use.
8. Demonstrate correct technique for changing tracheostomy tube.
9. State principles of skin care.
10. State precautions to be taken when outdoors.
11. Demonstrate proper feeding techniques.
12. State signs of illness, respiratory assessment.
13. State actions to be taken in event of tracheostomy obstruction, decannulation, and bleeding.
14. Demonstrate CPR.

and do not detect bradycardia. Parents must also be aware of the need to protect the child from the danger of aspiration of water or inhalation of cigarette smoke or other substances. They are instructed in emergency procedures and travel precautions (Table 10).

Because bath time is a particularly enjoyable time for babies, parents need suggestions on how to make bath time a *safe* time. We recommend using a very small amount of water (about one inch) and uninterrupted vigilance by the parents.

## Discharge

The child is usually discharged in the middle of the week, following completion of caretaker training. The attending pulmonologist contacts the local pediatrician several days prior to discharge to provide current information. A hospital discharge summary is mailed to the local doctor, and a copy is given to the parents. Children are transported to the home in the family automobile or van; we discourage the use of ambulance transport except in an emergency. Parents may be accompanied by a home care nurse if they find it is necessary; otherwise, the nurse meets them in the home. We recommend that families of continuously ventilated children have assisted caretaker support (volunteer or nurse) 24 hours per day for the first 2 weeks, then 16 hours per day for 2–4 weeks, then decrease as needed, usually to 12 hours per day.

**TABLE 11 ■ Rehospitalization of Riley HMV Patients with BPD**

| Patient# | Total Time on HMV* | Days Rehospitalized | # Rehospitalizations | %Time Rehospitalized | Reason for Admission |
|---|---|---|---|---|---|
| 15 | 14 months | 35 | 7 | 6.7 | Treatment of pulmonary exacerbations, bronchiolitis |
| 17 | 6 months | 0 | 0 | 0 | |
| 19 | 5 months | 65 | 2 | 43 | Treatment of pulmonary exacerbations, bronchiolitis |
| 20 | 3 months | 0 | 0 | 0 | |
| 22 | 2 1/2 years | 10 | 3 | .3 | Treatment of pulmonary exacerbations, bronchiolitis |

*Home mechanical ventilation

Children return to the pulmonary clinic at regular one- to two-month intervals, depending on their needs. At each visit, a thorough respiratory evaluation is performed along with multisystem assessment. Particular attention is paid to potential problems of chronic illness and immobility such as skin irritation or breakdown, constipation, urinary retention, inadequate positioning, and nutrition. The multidisciplinary team meets with the family to assess the program of care and the family's adjustment and to determine if alterations are indicated.

## Weaning

Weaning may not be possible for every ventilator-dependent child. Some children have progressive disease that precludes a decrease in ventilator support. Weaning from mechanical ventilation is a long-awaited milestone, however, for an infant with BPD. Unfortunately, the criteria for readiness to wean and weaning protocols are not well defined.

In an attempt to identify clinical correlates of successful weaning, Morray and coworkers studied seven hospitalized infants with BPD. They identified three stages of BPD: the "early phase," the "turning point," and the "actual weaning." The turning point, which signalled readiness to wean, was characterized by a decrease in respiratory rate, a decrease in arterial carbon dioxide tension, and improved average monthly weight gain.[6] We have incorporated these findings into our general weaning criteria, with the added restriction that the child must be free of respiratory infection currently and during the preceding two months.

Even if a child meets the weaning criteria, other problems may arise. If the process is to take place in the home, more personnel, increased observation time, and additional equipment are necessary. Many durable medical equipment vendors in our area supply ventilators and provide excellent service for them, but oximeters and end-tidal carbon dioxide monitors, both necessary for weaning, were not readily available for home rental until recently. In addition, some home ventilators may not accommodate the rate and volume changes necessary for weaning. Thus, the effort must be made to obtain a hospital ventilator for use in the home.

Four patients in our program have been weaned from mechanical ventilation (Table 1). The first child who was weaned had a chest wall abnormality secondary to renal osteodystophy; the weaning process took place in the hospital. The other three children were weaned at home.

We begin by decreasing the ventilator rate during awake periods by one breath per minute every two to three weeks. Ventilation and oxygenation are assessed by oximetry and end-tidal $CO_2$ monitoring during active and resting periods. In addition, heart rate, respiratory rate and effort, color, appetite, and general mood are carefully noted.

When the child has been weaned from daytime support, we wait one to two months for stabilization and then begin to wean during sleep time. Weaning from oxygen is the final step. It also takes place in stages—waking time first, then sleep time, ensuring that the child can maintain oxygen saturation greater than or equal to 90 percent in room air.

## Conclusion

Despite significant disease resulting in ventilator dependence, most children in our program have required minimal rehospitalization. The 20 current patients in our program have had a total of 60 rehospitalizations, amounting to 588 days; this accounts for 2.2 percent of their home mechanical ventilation time as a group. (For data on rehospitalization of patients with BPD, see Table 11.)

In the event of an emergency, the parents arrange for transport of the child to the nearest emergency facility, such as a community hospital. After assessment and stabilization, transfer to Riley Hospital can take place. For well-child care and nonemergency illnesses, such as gastroenteritis and otitis media, the child is seen by the primary care physician in the local community. Many physicians have found it easiest to make a house call for such visits, and parents certainly appreciate this alternative.

Although the stresses of caring for the chronically ill, technologically dependent child are numerous, we agree with other home care centers that this stress must be assessed *relative* to that imposed by prolonged hospitalization in an intensive care unit. Our families' anecdotal reports of the benefits of home care concur with those presented in the literature.[1,7-9] However, we recognize that home care may not be the most beneficial choice for every family and are working to develop alternative care strategies, such as extended care facilities and independent living centers, within the state of Indiana.

## Acknowledgement

The author would like to thank the parents of ventilator-dependent children who assisted in the development of this program.

## References

1. Burr BH, et al.: Home care for children on respirators, New England Journal of Medicine 309(21), 1983, p. 1319.
2. Goldberg AI: Home care for life-supported persons: Is a national approach the answer? Chest 90, 1986, pp. 744–748.
3. Goldberg AI et al.: Home care for life-supported persons: An approach to program development, Journal of Pediatrics 104(5), 1984, pp. 785–795.
4. Garay RM, et al.: Sustained reversal of chronic hypercapnia in patients with alveolar hypoventilation syndromes, American Journal of Medicine 63, 1977, p. 223.
5. Woollam CHM: The development of apparatus for intermittent negative pressure respiration, Anaesthesia 31, 1976, pp. 537–547, 666–685.
6. Morray JP, et al.: Improvement in lung mechanics as a function of age in the infant with severe bronchopulmonary dysplasia, Pediatric Research 16, 1982, pp. 290–294.
7. Frates RC, et al.: Outcome of home mechanical ventilation in children, Journal of Pediatrics 106(5), 1985, p. 850.
8. Schraeder BD: A creative approach to caring for the ventilator dependent child, The American Journal of Maternal-Child Nursing 4, 1979, p. 165.
9. Schreiner MS, et al.: Pediatric home mechanical ventilation, Pediatric Clinics of North America 34(1), 1987, pp. 47–60.

## Bibliography

- Children with handicaps and their families: Case example: the ventilator-dependent child. Report of the Surgeon General's Workshop, DHHS Publ. No. PHS-83-50194. Washington, DC, Department of Health and Human Services, 1983.
- Hartsell M, and Ward J: Selecting equipment vendors for children on home care, The American Journal of Maternal-Child Nursing 10(1), 1985, pp. 26–28.
- Olson D, and Henig E, eds.: Whatever happened to the polio patient? Proceedings of the First International Post Polio Conference, Rehabilitation Institute of Chicago/ March of Dimes, Chicago, 1981.

- Schreiner M, Donar M, and Kettrick R: Pediatric home mechanical ventilation, Pediatric Clinics of North America 34(1), 1987, pp. 47–60.
- Steele N, and Harrison B: Technology assisted children: Assessing discharge preparation, Journal of Pediatric Nursing 1, 1986, pp. 150–158.

# APPENDIX A

## Standardized Patient Care Plan for the Infant with Bronchopulmonary Dysplasia

*Lauren Thorngate, RN, MS, and*
*Barbera Herzog, RN, MS*
*Intensive Care Nursery*
*Children's Hospital, Oakland, California*

Bronchopulmonary dysplasia is a form of chronic lung disease. It is caused by ongoing injury and repair of lung tissue. Hypoxic injury to an immature lung is exacerbated by high inspired oxygen tensions and barotrauma related to mechanical ventilation and infection. It is diagnosed and classified into stages of severity by radiographic changes, differences in pulmonary function, and clinical presentation.

**Target population:** Infants requiring assisted ventilation for more than one month

| DATE | NURSING DIAGNOSIS/PROBLEM | EXPECTED OUTCOMES | NURSING PLAN | STATUS OF NURSING DIAGNOSIS/PROBLEM | NURSE INITIALS |
|---|---|---|---|---|---|
| | ***Actual or Potential*** | | | | |
| | 1. Alterations in nutrition: less than body requirements due to increased caloric need and restricted fluid intake | Infant will maintain adequate caloric need intake as evidenced by:<br>a. weight gain of 10–30 gm/day<br>b. appropriate increase in head circumference and length<br>By (date) ________<br>During hospitalization ___<br>Before discharge______ | a. Maintain caloric intake records<br>b. Monitor measurements of weight, head circumference, and length<br>c. Utilize calorically dense solutions; increase glucose, increase % intralipids, 24 kcal/oz formula<br>d. Consult dietitian for age-appropriate nutrition (solids) | | |
| | 2. Alteration in nutrition: less than body requirements due to feeding intolerance | Infant will tolerate feedings as evidenced by:<br>a. no emesis or residual<br>b. stable abdominal girth<br>By (date) ________<br>During hospitalization ___<br>Before discharge______ | a. Plan care around feeding schedule<br>b. Give bolus gavage feedings slowly, and when infant calm<br>c. Routinely check residuals; report significant changes<br>d. Consider long-term polyurethane NG tubes.<br>e. Monitor stooling pattern and heme test stool as ordered<br>f. Position on abdomen or side after feedings | | |

| | | | | |
|---|---|---|---|---|
| 3. Alterations in nutrition due to inability to retain feedings secondary to gastroesophageal reflux | Infant will retain feedings without emesis.<br>By (date) ____<br>During hospitalization ____<br>Before discharge ____ | a. Record and report emesis<br>b. Elevate head of bed<br>c. Individualize positioning per baby's response | | |
| **COLLABORATIVE PROBLEM:**<br>***Actual or Potential***<br>4. Electrolyte imbalance | Infant will maintain adequate fluid and electrolyte balance as evidenced by:<br>a. good skin turgor<br>b. adequate blood pressure<br>c. normal pulse<br>d. well-hydrated mucous membranes<br>By (date) ____<br>During hospitalization ____<br>Before discharge ____ | a. Monitor electrolyte levels, as ordered, especially if on diuretic therapy<br>b. Check specific gravity readings as ordered<br>c. Administer electrolyte and formula additives as ordered<br>d. Assess for signs of electrolyte depletion:<br>—hydration<br>—blood pressure<br>—pulse<br>—muscle tone<br>—twitching | | |
| 5. Injury due to osteopenia secondary to alterations in nutrition | Absence of fractures<br>By (date) ____<br>During hospitalization ____<br>Before discharge ____ | a. Administer gentle range of motion and body alignment<br>b. Observe limbs and joints for unusual posture<br>c. Observe infant for excessive crying upon | | |

| Date | Nursing Diagnosis/Problem | Expected Outcomes | Nursing Plan | Status of Nursing Diagnosis/Problem | Nurse Initials |
|---|---|---|---|---|---|
| | | | movement<br>d. Administer gentle postural drainage as ordered<br>e. Alert staff through use of "Handle with Care" signs at bedside<br>f. Monitor calcium and phosphorus levels as ordered | | |
| | 6. Alterations in respiratory functions due to impaired gas exchange | Blood gases will demonstrate acceptable gas exchange.<br>By (date) ______________<br>During hospitalization ___<br>Before discharge________ | a. Increase $FiO_2$ to maintain oxygenation during feeding, crying, suctioning, or blood drawing<br>b. Minimize hypoxic episodes<br>c. Allow adequate rest periods; document recovery time after procedures<br>d. Monitor and record gas exchange; document with ABGs, TCM, oximetry<br>e. Consider use of lidocaine with peripheral ABGs, per protocol | | |

| | | | | |
|---|---|---|---|---|
| 7. Alterations in respiratory function due to potential for reactive airway or bronchospasm. | Decreased occurrence of bronchospasm<br>By (date) ______<br>During hospitalization ___<br>Before discharge______ | a. Assess breath sounds for equality, aeration, chest expansion<br>b. Consider hand ventilation with adjusted pressure and I time<br>c. Keep ventilator tubing free of excess water to decrease risk of aspiration<br>d. Assess for specific precipitating events; document<br>e. Utilize aerosol and/or systemic bronchodilators as ordered<br>f. Decrease stress reaction through use of sedation as ordered; document effect | | |
| 8. Alterations in respiratory function due to potential for pulmonary edema | Infant will demonstrate:<br>a. clear breath sounds<br>b. stable weights<br>c. adequate gas exchange<br>By (date) ______<br>During hospitalization ___<br>Before discharge______ | a. Obtain daily weights; report significant changes (an increase above 30 gm)<br>b. Monitor strict I&O<br>c. Assess breath sounds for quality of aeration; report changes<br>d. Position on abdomen frequently with head elevated<br>e. Observe for signs of | | |

| Date | Nursing Diagnosis/Problem | Expected Outcomes | Nursing Plan | Status of Nursing Diagnosis/Problem | Nurse Initials |
|---|---|---|---|---|---|
| | | | edema:<br>—rales<br>—decreased output<br>—periorbital and genital edema<br>f. Administer diuretics as ordered<br>g. Individualize weaning from assisted ventilation | | |
| | 9. Alterations in sensory perception due to environmental stimuli | Infant will be protected from stimulation as evidenced by adequate rest periods.<br>By (date) ______<br>During hospitalization ___<br>Before discharge ______ | a. Reduce light at bedside; shield patient's eyes<br>b. Keep bedside area quiet<br>c. Observe toleration level of procedures and recovery time; document<br>d. Individualize care based on response to stimuli<br>e. Alert staff and family to need for minimal handling<br>f. Request consult with child development specialist for individual care | | |

| | | | | |
|---|---|---|---|---|
| 10. Delayed development due to hospitalization and fragile state | Infant will achieve optimal growth and development.<br>By (date) ________<br>During hospitalization ___<br>Before discharge________ | a. Observe infant for times of calm alertness and utilize these times to introduce stimulation<br>b. Provide for consistency of caretakers as much as possible<br>c. Consult child development specialist to develop an individualized approach, including:<br>—visual stimulation<br>—audio stimulation<br>—tactile stimulation<br>—social stimulation<br>d. Observe for signs of hearing or vision impairment and document | | |
| 11. Alteration in parenting due to interruption of parenting role and family interaction | a. Parents will develop strong bonding relationships.<br>b. Parents will be actively involved in care.<br>By (date) ________<br>During hospitalization ___<br>Before discharge________ | a. Encourage parents and family to visit and call<br>b. Assist parents in recognizing and understanding cues for tolerating stimulation:<br>—physiological changes (vital signs, pulse oximeter, TCM)<br>—color change<br>—level of activity<br>c. Encourage and assist parents in touching and | | |

| DATE | NURSING DIAGNOSIS/PROBLEM | EXPECTED OUTCOMES | NURSING PLAN | STATUS OF NURSING DIAGNOSIS/PROBLEM | NURSE INITIALS |
|---|---|---|---|---|---|
| | | | holding their baby<br>d. Work with social workers to assist parents in contacting parent support groups and buddies<br>e. Assist in coordination of family-staff conferences<br>f. Assist parents in evaluating needs; teach on a day-to-day basis; document response<br>g. Encourage parents to keep track of infant's progress with photographs<br>h. Encourage parents to select appropriate toys and clothing<br>i. Involve parents in infant's care when appropriate<br>j. Allow parents and family to freely express fears, anxiety, and concerns<br>k. Communicate specific parental needs to social workers<br>l. Identify back-up caretaker and involve in | | |

| | | | | |
|---|---|---|---|---|
| | | discharge teaching<br>m. Develop and implement a discharge teaching plan | | |
| 12. Alteration in sleep pattern due to inability to initiate self-comforting measures | Infant will achieve adequate daily rest.<br>By (date) ______<br>During hospitalization ____<br>Before discharge ______ | a. Utilize calming techniques:<br>—patting<br>—swaddling<br>—holding<br>—electric fan<br>b. Change position prn, preferably to sidelying or prone<br>c. Support body alignment with blanket rolls and sandbags, or swaddle<br>d. Offer comfort measures after invasive procedures to foster trust<br>e. Follow individual plan of care; document response<br>f. Alert caretakers to most effective approaches through signs and documentation at bedside; update as needed | | |

| Date | Nursing Diagnosis/Problem | Expected Outcomes | Nursing Plan | Status of Nursing Diagnosis/Problem | Nurse Initials |
|---|---|---|---|---|---|
| | 13. Infection due to immature immune system and number of invasive procedures | a. Vital signs will be maintained within normal limits.<br>b. Absence of clinical signs of infection<br>By (date) ______<br>During hospitalization ___<br>Before discharge______ | a. Assess and document clinical signs of infection:<br>—perfusion<br>—lethargy<br>—apnea/bradycardia<br>—temperature instability<br>—feeding intolerance<br>—irritability<br>b. Monitor vital signs<br>c. Use meticulous hand washing<br>d. Maintain sterile technique for ETT suctioning<br>e. Screen visitors and caretakers for possible infection<br>f. Use aseptic technique for all invasive procedures including indwelling lines or catheters<br>g. Position on abdomen during and after feeding to prevent aspiration | | |

# APPENDIX B

## Guidelines for the Care of an Extubated Infant

*Roslyn Feller Scherf, RNC*

| Problem | Goals of Therapy | Actions |
|---|---|---|
| ***Pulmonary*** | | |
| **1. Infant Becomes $O_2$ Dependent:** | | |
| Prolonged high inspired oxygen levels destroy existing Type I cells and are replaced with poorly functioning Type II alveolar cells. | The amount of time an infant is $O_2$ dependent varies.<br>In general, $FiO_2$ will be weaned as the infant's weight increases and as lungs and airways begin to grow and develop. | When an infant is $O_2$ dependent, maintain required $FiO_2$ at all times and especially during periods of stress such as crying when blood work is drawn, while starting an IV, during an LP, suctioning, chest physiotherapy (CPT), feeding, and so forth. (Also see actions under Psychosocial Development.)<br>At times, $FiO_2$ may even need to be temporarily increased during some of these procedures if they cause hypoxemia. Monitoring $TcPO_2$ or pulse oximetry ($SaO_2$) may also be helpful during these procedures. |
| Inflammation and destruction of the alveolar wall or of its capillary bed leads to a destructive form of emphysema. Because of the airlessness or collapse of some alveoli, and the overinflation of other alveoli, parts of the vascular bed are condensed in the scarring that occurs. The capillaries are separated from alveolar spaces, and the vascular bed is reduced in volume. In the aerated regions, the arteries grow but receive an abnormally large part of the cardiac output.[10,15,19] Therefore, large portions of the capillary bed must remodel the damaged lung. A diffusion barrier is now created, leading to an inability to decrease $FiO_2$. | Improvements in pulmonary function tests will occur if the infant is growing.<br>Respiratory rate, retractions, and nasal flaring will decrease, or at least not increase, when $FiO_2$ is decreased.<br>Acceptable limits for $PaO_2$: Arterial = 50–70 mmHg (and sometimes 80 mmHg) and capillary = 40–60 mmHg. An infant with multiple problems (weight gain or cor pulmonale) might require a higher $PaO_2$. | Make sure a capillary blood gas (CBG) or arterial blood gas (ABG) is done according to the chronic blood gas protocol (for our unit, every 3 days or 20 minutes after a permanent change in $FiO_2$ is made) and more frequently if the infant shows signs of distress such as an increased respiratory rate, increased heart rate, cyanosis, increased retractions (subcostal and intercostal), rales, or lethargy.<br>Maintain $PaO_2$ within normal limits. Institute a weaning care plan. |
| On room air, hypoxemia, with its additional problems, can occur. | An acceptable limit for $PaCO_2$ is 45 mmHg up to 60 mmHg. (In some cases, higher $PaCO_2$ levels must be accepted, depending upon each infant's degree of illness and history. There are some infants with $PaCO_2$ levels in the high 60s who remain extubated | Maintain infant's normal body temperature, (Hypothermia and hyperthermia increase $O_2$ consumption and may increase $O_2$ requirements.)<br>Maintain adequate nutrition, which may help in the formation of new alveoli and enlargement of the diameter of the airways. This may result in an increase in lung compliance, a decrease in pulmonary |

| | | |
|---|---|---|
| | or continue to be weaned from the ventilator.) | resistance, and a better distribution of ventilation. The regression of fibrosis will help recovery. |
| **2. $CO_2$ Retention**<br>The retention of $CO_2$ is associated with an insufficient alveolar ventilation; it is probably the result of an increased dead space ventilation resulting from a small tidal volume.<br>**a. Decreased functional residual capacity: (sometimes FRC is normal or elevated.)**<br>This is probably secondary to the poorly ventilated areas of lung.<br>**b. Decreased compliance:**<br>Pressure damage can occur, especially to conducting airways and supporting tissues in alveolar junctional areas. The lung becomes increasingly stiff and overdistended. This results in a decreased tidal volume that, in turn, causes an increase in respiratory rate. (Tachypnea compensates for the small tidal volume.)<br>**c. Increased airway resistance:**<br>Bronchiolar necrosis, squamosis metaplasia, and eosinophilic exudate cause obstruction of the small bronchi. There is cellular | As he gains weight, the infant will begin to show improvements in pulmonary function tests.<br>$PaCO_2$ will decrease to an acceptable range (35–45 mm Hg). In some cases, however, a higher $PaCO_2$ is acceptable.<br>The infant will have a decrease in respiratory rate, a decrease or absence of subcostal and intercostal retractions, and a decrease or absence of nasal flaring and rales. | Postural drainage with CPT and vibration followed by suctioning should be done as needed. The frequency depends on the individual infant, the severity of the disease, and the degree of $CO_2$ retention, as shown by ABG or CBG. Increases in respiratory rate, retractions, rales, mucus, and/or atelectasis as observed on x-ray indicate a need for initiating or increasing the frequency of CPT.<br>However, allow rest periods as needed and make sure the therapy is not done too frequently, exhausting the infant.<br>Follow blood gases according to previously mentioned protocol and if an increase in respiratory rate or retractions occurs.<br>Maintain adequate nutrition and position infant on abdomen frequently. (Infants maintain a higher $TcPO_2$ and have improved ventilation when positioned on their abdomens.)<br>Prevent and minimize episodes of hypoxia as much as possible; that is, maintain required $FiO_2$ when starting IVs. |

| Problem | Goals of Therapy | Actions |
|---|---|---|
| proliferation both of epithelial layers and of connective tissue with excessive collagen production. As a result, hypertrophy of peribronchiolar smooth muscles occurs. | | |
| **d. Increased effort to breathe:** Due to a stiff, poorly compliant lung, the infant must use a lot of effort with each breath to overcome the resistance and stiffness. | | |
| **3. Complications of BPD** | | |
| **a. Atelectasis:** Atelectasis may be due to a plug of mucus. The blood in the capillaries rapidly absorbs the air in the entrapped alveoli, causing collapse of the alveoli. It frequently involves the left lower lobe, especially with an enlarged heart that compresses the left lower lobe bronchus. | After the diagnosis is made, improvement will be observed as soon as therapy is initiated. The lung will be fully expanded when the next x-ray is taken (usually within 12–24 hours).<br>The infant will have a decrease in respiratory rate, heart rate, retractions, and $PaCO_2$.<br>Breath sounds will improve, and the infant will be more active and alert. | Check breath sounds q 3–4 hours. Report changes immediately to physician.<br>Observe for (and report immediately) increases in respiratory rate, retractions, heart rate, cyanosis, lethargy, or readily tiring (especially with feedings).<br>Follow $PaCO_2$ via blood gases (per unit protocol).<br>Make sure chest x-rays are done, as ordered by physician.<br>Do CPT as ordered, concentrating on the left lower lobe and/or other atelectatic areas seen on x-ray.<br>Some infants may improve their ventilation if CPT and suctioning are followed by bag-mask ventilation for 2–5 minutes. If this is ordered, (1) make sure an OG tube is inserted into the stomach to allow air to escape (& prevent distension); (2) make sure the |

| | | |
|---|---|---|
| | | hand-ventilation is done with the infant properly positioned (not head flexed and occluding the trachea); (3) Monitor $TcPO_2$ or $SaO_2$ to detect if the infant becomes more hypoxic during the procedure. If he does, the order should be re-evaluated.; (4) make sure it is not done so frequently that the infant becomes totally exhausted.<br>Assist the physician with endotracheal suctioning whenever necessary.<br>Position the infant on his abdomen as much as possible. |
| **b. Pulmonary edema:**<br>Pulmonary edema is the result of excessive quantities of fluid in the alveoli or pulmonary interstitial spaces.<br>An increase in systemic vascular pressures could impair lymphatic drainage into the great veins, which, in turn, could enhance fluid accumulation in the lung.<br>Increased vascular permeability resulting in increased fluid in lung tissue can also occur. | The infant will be breathing more easily with a decrease in respiratory rate, heart rate, and retractions.<br>If present, bloody secretions will cease; amount of mucus obtained with suctioning will decrease.<br>Chest x-ray will improve.<br>Infant will be more active and alert.<br>If diuretics are given, a decrease in weight (30 or more grams) will be noted.<br>The diuretics we use frequently are:<br>1. Lasix (furosemide): 1–2 mg/kg/dose q 8–12 hr (occasionally q 6 hr), IV or PO or<br>2. Aldactone (spironolactone): | Avoid stressing the infant as this will increase his work of breathing. Some signs of stress include increased heart rate, cyanosis, lethargy, and extremely fussy and irritable behavior.<br>Closely monitor fluid intake and urine output—maintain an accurate record of intake and output as ordered by physician.<br>If fluids must be further restricted, check to see if a higher calorie formula can be given. If so, this will help maintain calories while decreasing fluid intake.<br>Weigh the infant daily and report any increase above 30 grams to physician.<br>Avoid bolus infusions (more than 10 cc/kg/hr) of IV fluids.<br>Administer blood transfusions over a 3–4 hr period (to avoid overloading the circulatory system).<br>Monitor respiratory rate and heart rate q 3–4 hr. Report any increase in respiratory rate, heart rate, and retractions to physician. Also, observe closely for an |

| Problem | Goals of Therapy | Actions |
|---|---|---|
| | 3 mg/kg/day q 12 hrs, PO or<br>3. Diuril (chlorothiazide): 10–40 mg/kg/day q 6–12 hrs, PO<br>Occasionally Aldactone and Diuril or Lasix and Diuril are given alternatingly on the same day (that is, Lasix $12^N$ and $12^M$, Diuril $6^A$ and $6^P$ or Aldactone $12^N$ and $12^M$, Diuril $6^A$ and $6^P$). | increase in secretions obtained when suctioning (especially if they are blood-tinged), cyanosis, presence or increase in rales, decrease in breath sounds, or lethargy. Report any of the above to the physician.<br>Elevate the head of the bed; position the infant on his abdomen frequently, monitor blood gases per protocol; and administer diuretics as ordered. |
| **c. Cor pulmonale:**<br>Cor pulmonale is also caused by the previously mentioned problems of pulmonary edema, as well as by right ventricular hypertrophy resulting in right-sided heart failure.<br>Extreme parenchymal disease and chronic hypoxia can lead to pulmonary hypertension. This can also contribute to right-sided heart failure. | Signs of fluid retention, such as:<br>• edema<br>• weight gain<br>• oliguria<br>• increased respiratory rate and/or heart rate<br>• increased $FiO_2$ requirements<br>• pulmonary edema will not be present.<br>On x-ray, heart size will decrease and lungs will show improvement.<br>$FiO_2$ requirements will stabilize or even decrease.<br>Decrease in tachypnea, rales, tachycardia, and retractions will occur.<br>The infant will be more alert and active. | Place on very strict intake and output and monitor closely. (Especially monitor IV infusion rates closely.) Check and record intake and output every hour. Report oliguria or diuresis to physician. Report excessive intake to physician, should it occur.<br>Elevate the head of the bed and place the infant in a position that seems to be the most comfortable for him.<br>Avoid frequent episodes of stress. Allow the infant to rest as frequently as needed.<br>Sedation with medications such as chloral hydrate, phenobarbital, etc., may be helpful.<br>Gavage rather than nipple feed (unless, with older babies, gavaging is more stressful).<br>Make sure blood gases are done as frequently as needed. If possible, try to monitor infant with a $TcPO_2$ or $SaO_2$ monitor, which is less stressful.<br>Institute a "minimal touch" policy by which you organize all care (nursing, respiratory, laboratory, and so forth) |

| | |
|---|---|
| Blood gases will be within normal limits. | so the infant is disturbed as little as possible. Limit the amount of care to prevent tiring the infant as much as possible. |
| If diuretics are given, a decrease in weight (30 or more grams) will be noted. | Place the infant on a cardiorespiratory monitor. Check heart rate, respiratory rate, breath sounds, and temperature at least q 3 hrs and blood pressure q 8–12 hrs. Maintain temperature according to the unit's thermoregulation policy. Report significant changes immediately to physician. |
| | If the infant is sleeping, heart rate,and respiratory rate may be taken from the monitor. (The frequency of vital signs applies only to the infant in cor pulmonale. He should be checked frequently but not necessarily awakened. If signs are taken from the monitor, the infant could possibly sleep for 5–6 hours. However, observe the infant closely and frequently). |
| | Temperature can sometimes be checked with the next set of vital signs, allowing the infant to sleep for several hours. (If the infant is hypothermic or hyperthermic, he will increase his $O_2$ consumption and might require an increase in $FiO_2$). |
| | Weigh at least every day and report immediately any weight gain above 30 grams. |
| | Observe for signs of fluid retention: excessive weight gain (>30 gm/day); edema, especially of the eyelids, genital areas (scrotum or labia), and lower extremities; increased respiratory rate; rales. |
| | Because fluids are usually restricted, also observe for signs of dehydration: depressed fontanel, decreased skin turgor, decreased urine output, increased urine specific gravity, and weight loss( >30 gm/day). |
| | For severe fluid restrictions check to see if a higher |

| Problem | Goals of Therapy | Actions |
|---|---|---|
| | | calorie formula can be given. |
| | | In more severe cases of dehydration, a decrease in blood pressure can be observed as well as an increase in lethargy and, at times, an increase in irritability. |
| | | Administer blood transfusions over at least 3–4 hrs to avoid overloading the circulatory system. Maintaining an adequate hematocrit (30–40 mg%) will provide the infant with an optimum oxygen carrying capacity. |
| | | Avoid bolus IV infusions (>10 cc/kg/hr). |
| | | Administer digoxin and diuretics as ordered. Make sure electrolytes such as $Na^+$ and $K^+$ are checked q 1–2 days while on digoxin and diuretics. However, in some cases electrolytes may need to be monitored more frequently, for example, if a large amount of diuresis occurs, if arrhythmias occur, or if there is a change in the dosages of the medications. |
| | | Be aware that the infant may require a $K^+$ supplement during therapy with diuretics. |
| | | Care is similar to that for infants with pulmonary edema. |

| | | |
|---|---|---|
| **d. Lower respiratory infections:**<br>Lower respiratory infections can be common during the first year of life. Some infections can be related to aspiration of feedings. | Secretions obtained with suctioning will decrease and be thinner and clearer.<br><br>Infant will breathe more easily, and there will be decreases in respiratory rate and retractions.<br><br>Chest x-ray will show improvement.<br><br>Infant's temperature will be within normal limits. | Administer antibiotics as ordered by physician.<br><br>Frequency of CPT with suctioning may need to be increased.<br><br>Closely observe the infant for any signs of gastric reflux or aspiration, i.e. coughing, increased respiratory distress, wheezing, or vomiting. Use extremely good hand-washing techniques and other measures to prevent cross-contamination. |
| **e. PDA:**<br>A PDA causes excessive pulmonary blood flow, resulting in pulmonary congestion. Also, excessive fluid intake can aggravate the left heart failure in patients with a PDA and possibly increase the risk of developing BPD and/or aggravate the problems associated with BPD. | The signs of PDA will be readily identified and treatment will be rapidly initiated.<br><br>Improvement or disappearance of the signs of a PDA will be noted within 24 hours of initiating treatment.*<br><br>$FiO_2$ requirements will decrease as the PDA becomes less significant.<br><br>Closure of the PDA.<br><br>*Signs of PDA:<br>Heart murmur,active precordium, bounding pulses, cardiomegaly on x-ray, pulmonary edema, hepatomegaly, increasing $FiO_2$ requirements, increased respiratory rate and increased heart rate, excessive weight gain | Check vital signs at least every 3–4 hours during the first 28 days of life. As the infant grows older and remains stable, vital signs can be taken less frequently at night to allow him to sleep.<br><br>Avoid excessive fluid intake, especially IV bolus injections. Record intake and output.<br><br>Administer blood transfusions over a 3–4 hour period.<br><br>Weigh daily.<br><br>Observe for signs of a PDA and report them to the physician immediately.<br><br>If indomethacin is to be given, perform pre-indomethicin blood work and confer with physician when the results are available.<br><br>Observe for the side effects of indomethicin, that is, oliguria, vomiting, abdominal distension, prolonged bleeding.<br><br>Observe closely for signs of cor pulmonale. |

| Problem | Goals of Therapy | Actions |
|---|---|---|
| | and/or edema, and increased $PaCO_2$ (shown by blood gases). (In our unit, usually two or more of these signs must be present to make the diagnosis of a PDA.) | |
| ***Nutrition*** | | |
| Maintain adequate nutrition. Feeding intolerance can be common, and frequently the infant is on fluid restriction.<br>Due to the increased work of breathing, the infant has an increase in caloric expenditure.<br>Growth failure is common.<br>Adequate nutrition is needed for the formation of new alveoli and enlargement of the diameter of the airways. Oxygen consumption increases during feedings. | The infant will gain 10–30 grams per day. (This refers to an appropriate weight gain, not edema or "flabby fat.")<br>Head circumference and length will increase according to regular growth scales.<br>As the infant grows, pulmonary function tests will show improvements, that is, an increase in compliance and an improvement in functional residual capacity.<br>$FiO_2$ requirements will gradually decrease until he is on room air and remains on room air. | If at all possible, make sure the infant receives at least 90 cal/kg/day, increasing caloric intake daily until reaching at least 130 cal/kg/day.<br>If the infant is NPO, check with the physician to see if PHAF and/or lipids can be given.<br>If tolerated, give 24 calorie formula as soon as possible (especially if the infant is on fluid restrictions).<br>Depending upon each unit's feeding protocol, polycose or MCT oil can also be added to feedings. For the older infant, cereal can be added at 2 months of age, and fruits and vegetables at 4–6 months of age.<br>For smaller infants, unless it is more stressful, gavage feed the infant most of the time until a steady weight gain is noted and respirations are easier and less labored. However, if he becomes too irritated with gavage feedings and PO feedings are less stressful, then PO feed.<br>In some cases, increase $FiO_2$ (by physician's orders) during feedings, particularly nipple feedings (especially if $TcPO_2$ shows a decrease during feedings into hypoxic ranges). (For a TC monitor that is recording accurately, a value equaling below a $PaO_2$ of 50 mm Hg is a significant decrease.) |

| | | |
|---|---|---|
| | | Maintain temperature according to thermoregulation policy.<br>Avoid stressing the infant.<br>Occasionally, if feeding schedule appears to be stressing the infant, smaller, more frequent feedings may be required.<br>Supplemental calcium or vitamin D may be required, especially for the infant with a limited formula intake.<br>Vitamin E can be given PO when the infant is tolerating PO or gavage feedings. However, the exact benefits of giving vitamin E prophylactically in relationship to the prevention or management of BPD is not fully known. |
| ***Plus:***<br>**a. Fractures:**<br>Fractures may be due to a dietary or parenteral alimentation deficiency of calcium or vitamin D.<br>There also may be a calciuric effect of chronic furosemide administration.<br>In addition, the infant could be especially susceptible to rib fractures caused by CPT. | Fractures, if present, will be readily detected and appropriate treatment will be instituted. | Observe closely for any signs of fractures: abnormal protrusions of bone, swelling of joints or other areas, excessive crying (as if in pain) when moving extremities or during CPT, shorter limb compared to opposite limb, or unnatural movement in an area that is normally rigid.<br>Make sure infant receives supplementary vitamin D, as ordered by physician. |

| Problem | Goals of Therapy | Actions |
|---|---|---|
| ***Interference with the Normal Psychosocial Development*** | | |
| The infant is isolated from the normal environment due to oxygen requirements and chronic, prolonged hospitalization. He has a lack of normal sensory stimulation and social interaction. | The infant will exhibit social skills such as eye contact, smiling, and so forth at the appropriate age for such skills or at least shortly afterwards. | Provisions for psychosensory stimulation must be made available whenever possible. |
| The infant is exposed to repeated painful or uncomfortable stimulation, that is, blood sampling, suctioning, frequent chest physiotherapy, NG feedings, and so forth. | He will develop gross motor skills appropriately. | During feeding, bathing, and CPT, the older infant (over 28 days) should have another oxygen source, such as a nasal cannula. This will enable him to have a more normal contact with the environment and the care provider. It will also allow eye contact to occur. |
| In older infants, practice of such gross motor skills, such as rolling over and sitting up, is limited. | The parents will feel the child does belong to them and is a part of their family. They will also feel they have some control over their infant's social and sensory development. | Large oxyhoods may be used and fitted around the infant's chest, with arms inside to allow for hand-to-mouth and hand-to-hand contact. |
| Recent data suggest that some infants with BPD have an increased incidence of developmental delays, and *some* have severe handicaps, that is, deafness, blindness, and cerebral palsy. | | Some visual stimulation is possible also. Pictures, toys, and music boxes may be placed in and around the incubator or crib and even on or in the oxyhood. |
| Another problem that can occur is interference in the maternal-infant bonding process. Emotional deprivation due to the severity of illness and the prolonged hospitalization | | A nasal cannula is especially useful in a stable, older infant who is developing gross motor skills and is too active for a hood or tent. It will also allow for increased interactions with the people caring for him. |
| | | Oxygen tubing should be long enough to allow the infant to move around. |
| | | Whenever possible, especially during feeding or bath time, play with the infant and talk to him. However, do not overly stress the infant. |
| | | A volunteer foster grandparent may be requested, especially if the parents are unable to (or do not) visit frequently. |
| | | The infant may also be referred to an infant-developmental intervention program, if one is |

| | | |
|---|---|---|
| compounds the problems of psychosocial development.<br>The parents may feel they have no control over their baby's developmental processes. Due to the severity of their infant's illness and his various complications, the parents may feel frightened and inadequate, or possibly angry and hostile. | | available. From the information provided, a program can be developed for the infant to provide optimal stimulation and development.<br>When parents do visit, encourage them to handle, talk to, and play with their infant. Refer to the infant by his first name, thus recognizing him as an individual person.<br>Also encourage the parents to bring in toys, pictures, and clothes for their infant.<br>Parents could also participate in the program developed for their infant by the infant educator. Allow the parents to express their fears, anxieties, and concerns about their infant. If necessary, arrange for meetings with physicians, nurses, and other staff members (infant stimulator) so the parents can obtain answers to their questions. |
| ***Discharge Planning***<br>The parents must be aware of specific needs their infant may have as a result of having BPD.<br>Some of these needs include:<br>1. Being aware the infant may tire more readily and allowing him to rest as needed.<br>2. The possibility of more frequent feedings to achieve an appropriate weight gain.<br>3. Decreasing, as much as possible, his contact with people who have upper respiratory | Parents will be well prepared to take their infant home and continue with his plan of care as outlined in the discharge planning sessions. | Instruct the parents to observe their infant's normal breathing pattern. Note depth and type of retractions, if present; normal resting color; color when he is fussy and crying; amount of time to return to normal color after crying episodes; rate of respirations; presence or absence of nasal flaring.<br>Encourage parents to keep the infant away from people who have colds or other respiratory infections because their infant will be prone to developing colds due to his lung disease.<br>If he develops a cold or respiratory infection, take the infant to his pediatrician or clinic to be examined.<br>Inform the parents that the infant may have some respiratory distress during a cold and to closely |

| Problem | Goals of Therapy | Actions |
|---|---|---|
| infections (URI). | | observe the infant for such distress. Call the physician if necessary. Inform parents of the possibility of rehospitalization, should his condition deteriorate. However, at the same time, reassure them that they have not failed in caring for their child should rehospitalization be required. |
| 4. His proneness to develop frequent colds and URIs and the need for immediate medical treatment of these problems. | | |
| 5. Frequent follow-up clinic appointments for other problems—RLF, rickets, and so forth. | | Frequent rest periods may be necessary at this time, especially during feedings. |
| 6. Possibly, extra time and patience required to care for the infant (that is, longer feeding times), and in the expectations of his growth and development (that is, a longer time to reach normal weight for his age group). | | Some hospitals do have programs available that enable infants on oxygen to be discharged to their homes, If such programs are available, parents can then be referred to them. For those infants going home, who still require oxygen therapy and/or ventilatory support, a very detailed plan of care should be developed. The parents should also be included in developing this plan of care. |
| | | Inform parents that even though their infant has BPD, there is an excellent chance for him to grow and develop as a normal child, although that development may be somewhat delayed. |
| | | Allow parents to ask questions and express their anxieties while also providing a way to answer and meet those questions and anxieties (that is, through follow-up clinic visits, visiting nurse calls, and discharge planning programs). |

# APPENDIX C

## The Neonatal Individualized Developmental Care and Assessment Program (NIDCAP)

### A Training Program for Health Care Professionals in Developmental Observation, Assessment, and Care of High-Risk Newborns

**Brigham and Women's Hospital**
75 Francis St.,
Boston, Massachusetts 02115

**Children's Hospital**
300 Longwood Ave.,
Boston, Massachusetts 02115

*Co-directors:*

Heideleise Als, PhD

Deborah M. Buehler, EdM

**Training Centers Outside Boston**

*NIDCAP Level I: Observational Training for Improved Caregiving*

**University Medical Center**
1501 North Campbell Ave., Tucson, AZ 85724
Trainers: Elsa Sell, MD, and Susann Hill, MA

**The University of Oklahoma, Oklahoma Infant Transition Program**
940 North 13th St. Rm. 3N-361 Oklahoma City, OK 73126
Trainer: Joy Voyles Browne, RN, MSN, PhD

**Child Development Center, Children's Hospital Medical Center**
747 52nd St., Oakland, California 94609
Trainers: Kathleen A. VandenBerg, MA, and Bette Flushman, MA

**Wake Medical Center, Wake AHEC, Pediatric Teaching**
3000 New Bern Avenue, Raleigh, NC 27610
Trainers: James M. Helm, PhD, and Ann Marie MacLeod, LPT

*NIDCAP Level II: APIB Training*

**Saguaro APIB Training Center, University Medical Center**
1501 No. Campbell Ave., Tucson Arizona 85724
Director: Elsa Sell, MD, Associate Professor of Pediatrics

# APPENDIX D

# Discharge Teaching Plan for the Infant with Bronchopulmonary Dysplasia

*Rose Jereb, BSN, and*
*Lauren Thorngate, RN, MS*
*Children's Hospital*
*Oakland, California*

| DATE | FAMILY MEMBER | RN | EXPECTED OUTCOMES | INTERVENTIONS | EVALUATION |
|---|---|---|---|---|---|
| **NURSING DIAGNOSIS: Knowledge Deficit of Bronchopulmonary Dysplasia** | | | | | |
| | | | ***Family will be able to:***<br>Discuss nature of the disease | ***Nurse will describe:***<br>Increased work of breathing due to:<br>stiffness of lungs<br>extra fluid<br>Chronic illness<br>require special care (especially first year)<br>possibility of rehospitalization | |
| | | | Discuss need for careful respiratory assessment | Importance of early recognition of respiratory compromise | |
| | | | Discuss need for medication | Function of diuretics, bronchodilators and electrolyte replacement | |
| | | | Discuss need for home oxygen | Increased $O_2$ needs due to increased work of breathing<br>Fluctuating needs due to stress, feeding or sleep | |
| | | | Discuss nutritional needs | Increased caloric needs and less energy due to increased work of breathing<br>Possible need for nutritional supplements:<br>Polycose, MCT oil, Breastmilk fortifier | |

| | | | | |
|---|---|---|---|---|
| | | Discuss potential for dehydration | Fluid and electrolyte loss related to:<br>diuretics<br>respiratory infection<br>fever | |
| | | Discuss potential for respiratory infection | Susceptibility for respiratory infection<br>Transmission of respiratory virus<br>coughing and sneezing<br>unwashed hands | |
| | | Discuss potential need for emergency measures | Purpose of home monitoring (if applicable)<br>Potential need for infant resuscitation:<br>Apnea detection/stimulation, CPR, choking<br>Need for emergency plan | |

**NURSING DIAGNOSIS: Alterations in Respiratory Function**

| | | | | |
|---|---|---|---|---|
| | | ***Family will demonstrate:***<br>Respiratory assessment | ***Nurse will explain and demonstrate:***<br>Counting respirations for one minute<br>Identification of retractions and work of breathing<br>Identification of color changes<br>Identification of wheezing, congestion, grunting and nasal flaring<br>Identification of apnea, periodic breathing and tachypnea<br>Identification of other signs of infection:<br>Loss of appetite, changes in behavior and sleeping patterns | |
| | | Identification of baseline respiratory status | At rest, during and after stress:<br>Respiratory rate<br>Quality of respirations | |

| DATE | FAMILY MEMBER | RN | EXPECTED OUTCOMES | INTERVENTIONS | EVALUATION |
|---|---|---|---|---|---|
| | | | | Skin color | |
| | | | Medication administration:<br>Draw up and administer<br>State when and how often | Use of syringe (tape to mark dose)<br>Ways to administer (mouth, nipple, bottle)<br>Use of medication calendar<br>Appropriate timing of doses<br>Side effects and signs of toxicity<br>Diuretics—dehydration/fluid overload<br>Theophylline—vomiting, irritability, tachycardia | |
| | | | Home oxygen administration:<br>Understanding of safety<br>Cannula taping<br>Mechanics of equipment<br>Ordered flow rate<br>Knowledge of supply needs | Fire hazard: smoking, open flame<br>Method of cannula taping<br>Schedule of changing (weekly, and as needed)<br>Check tubing: loose connections, crimping, excessive length<br>Check tank: level, on/off, flow rate<br>Delivery of flow rate: continuous, adjust only as ordered by MD<br>Check tank daily, anticipation of reorder | |

**NURSING DIAGNOSIS: Alterations in Nutrition: less than body requirements**

| | | | | | |
|---|---|---|---|---|---|
| | | | ***Family will be able to:***<br>Discuss adequate and optimal intake | ***Nurse will explain:***<br>Number of ounces per day<br>Adequate 100 kcal/kg/day<br>Optimal 120 kcal/kg/day (or higher)<br>(divide by caloric density i.e.: 24 kcal/oz formula)<br>Frequency of feeding<br>Adjust according to individual needs and average per feeding intake<br>Should not supplement formula with water unless directed by physician<br>Consult pediatrician for appropriate introduction of solids | |
| | | | Discuss technique for mixing formula | Recipe for higher calorie formula<br>Additions of nutritional supplements<br>Human milk fortifier, Polycose, MCT oil<br>Clean technique<br>Wash with hot soapy water<br>Dishwasher<br>Acceptable length of refrigeration—24 hrs | |
| | | | Demonstrate effective feeding technique | Proper positioning during and after feeding<br>Appropriate size and type of nipple<br>Appropriate cheek and chin support<br>Reducing distractions during feeding<br>Pacing during feeding<br>Intervals and techniques for burping<br>If breastfeeding, appropriate sucking pattern, assessment of intake, and use of supplements | |

| DATE | FAMILY MEMBER | RN | EXPECTED OUTCOMES | INTERVENTIONS | EVALUATION |
|---|---|---|---|---|---|
| **NURSING DIAGNOSIS: Alterations in Fluid and Electrolyte Balance** | | | | | |
| | | | ***Family will be able to:*** | ***Nurse will describe:*** | |
| | | | Discuss signs and symptoms of dehydration | Dry mucus membranes, decreased urine output sunken fontanele, lethargy, poor feeding, weight loss | |
| | | | Discuss signs of fluid overload | Edema (facial and extremity), lung congestion, change in urine output, excessive weight gain | |
| | | | Demonstrate administration of electrolyte replacement | Correct measurement<br>Addition to formula—mix with daily batch<br>Need for close follow-up | |
| **NURSING DIAGNOSIS: Alterations in Health Care Maintenance** | | | | | |
| | | | ***Family will be able to:*** | ***Nurse will explain and demonstrate:*** | |
| | | | Discuss optimal environment | Desirable environmental temperature<br>Avoid drafts<br>Keep room temperature comfortable<br>Dress appropriately<br>No smoking in the same room<br>Screen visitors for respiratory infection<br>Avoid crowded places | |

| | | | | |
|---|---|---|---|---|
| | | Discuss ways to minimize risk of respiratory infection | Good handwashing<br>Wash before contact<br>Avoid sneezing, coughing, touching nose during contact<br>Minimize exposure to small children | |
| | | Describe ongoing plan for follow-up | Need for involvement of various disciplines<br>OT/PT, audiology, pulmonary, developmental<br>Importance of keeping appointments<br>Group appointments together for ease of transportation<br>Function of PHN/neonatal follow up | |
| | | Devise and describe emergency plan | Completion of emergency phone list<br>Appropriate activation of the EMS (911)<br>Identification of additional emergency support (family, neighbors)<br>Importance of notifying pediatrician | |
| | | Demonstrate effective emergency measures and infant CPR if appropriate | Apnea detection and stimulation<br>Choking measures<br>Infant CPR<br>When to activate EMS during resuscitation<br>Back up support and caretakers<br>Procedure for successful secondary return demonstration<br>Encourage official certification through Red Cross, American Heart Association, Community Agencies | |
| | | Discuss meaning of home monitor alarms (if applicable) | Apnea—no breath for more than 20 seconds<br>Bradycardia—heart rate less than 80<br>Tachycardia—heart rate greater than 220 | |

| DATE | FAMILY MEMBER | RN | EXPECTED OUTCOMES | INTERVENTIONS | EVALUATION |
|---|---|---|---|---|---|
| | | | Discuss appropriate response to alarms | When alarm sounds:<br>1. Look at the infant checking for breathing and color (if needed, initiate emergency measures)<br>2. Look at the monitor to check alarm light<br>3. Record problem, notify pediatrician | |
| | | | Discuss proper use of monitor | Placement of monitor on hard, open surface check hearing distance, ability to respond within 10 seconds (vacuum cleaner, running water may mask sound)<br>When to use: always while asleep, may remove when holding, must remove for bath<br>Close supervision of siblings required<br>Check skin condition under belt daily<br>Wean only per pediatrician | |
| **NURSING DIAGNOSIS: Alterations in Development** | | | | | |
| | | | ***Family will be able to:***<br>Discuss potential for developmental delay | ***Nurse will:***<br>Describe delay due to prematurity and hospitalization<br>Emphasize the concept of corrected age<br>Encourage utilization of informative materials (Premature Baby Book, Prematurely Yours film) | |

| | | | | |
|---|---|---|---|---|
| | | Discuss developmental needs | Emphasize importance of close developmental follow-up for age appropriate stimulation<br><br>Describe behavioral cues: stress, pleasure, level of alertness<br>Assist family in identification of individual cues<br>Encourage stimulation based on response: allow for period of recovery<br>Allow for period of adjustment to home environment (light, sound, feeling of security) | |

**NURSING DIAGNOSIS: Alterations in Parenting**

| | | | | |
|---|---|---|---|---|
| | | ***Family will be able to:***<br>Develop healthy interactive relationship with infant | ***Nurse will:***<br>Describe need for extended visits to become familiar with care needs and behavior patterns<br>Assist family in assuming caregiving role<br>Provide family with privacy to promote interaction<br>Reinforce positive interactive behaviors<br>Assure family that time is necessary for development of rapport | |
| | | Verbalize parenting expectations and needs | Assist family in identifying perception of illness<br>How do you see your baby?<br>How will this affect your family?<br>Encourage family to express anxieties and concerns related to discharge and changes in lifestyle<br>Assist family to increase awareness of need for relief and proper rest | |

| DATE | FAMILY MEMBER | RN | EXPECTED OUTCOMES | INTERVENTIONS | EVALUATION |
|---|---|---|---|---|---|
| | | | | Assist family in identifying backup caregivers<br>Facilitate awareness of impact on siblings | |
| **NURSING DIAGNOSIS: Potential for Social Isolation** | | | | | |
| | | | ***Family will be able to:***<br>Identify available community resources | ***Nurse will:***<br>Facilitate family's assessment of support needs: respite, emotional, financial, transportation, supplies<br>Collaborate with social service to provide information regarding community support | |
| | | | Develop functional support network | Foster development of appropriate coping mechanisms<br>Assist family to identify personal support systems (friends, family, church, neighbors)<br>Encourage involvement in parent support groups | |

# Appendix E

# Home Ventilation Program:

## James Whitcomb Riley Hospital for Children

The James Whitcomb Riley Hospital Home Ventilator Program was established in 1976 to support children who require mechanical ventilation in their homes. Services are provided by the multidisciplinary pulmonary team, which includes physicians, nurses, social workers, respiratory therapists, occupational, physical, and speech therapists, nutritionists, and child psychologists. Children who require positive or negative pressure ventilation on a full-time or part-time basis are candidates for the program. The following services are provided:

- Family assessment of medical and psychosocial suitability for home ventilatory management
- Comprehensive discharge planning, with participation by inpatient and outpatient team members, including tertiary and primary caregivers
- Analysis of required care and investigation of sources of payment for home care equipment and personnel
- Pulmonary follow-up care for all program participants
- 24-hour availability of pediatric pulmonologist
- Supportive counseling for child and family
- Hospital-based education of individuals who will provide home care (family, volunteers and nurses)
- Periodic reevaluation of family situation after discharge

To promote multidisciplinary communication, planning, and implementation, the following responsibilities have been delineated:

### Physician Responsibilities:

1. Medical management and stabilization
2. Initial communication with parents regarding home ventilator program
3. Written order "begin home ventilator program"
4. Communication with primary care physician:
   –Initial
   –Update
   –Predischarge
5. Discharge summary ready to go with patient

### Pulmonary Nurse Specialist Responsibilities:

1. Schedule and coordinate all multidisciplinary meetings regarding home ventilation of patient
2. Review checklist with care team at initial meeting
3. Provide parents with overview of home ventilator program, explain roles of each team member, explain home care planning process
4. Plan and coordinate teaching program for parents and other caregivers, in collaboration with primary nurse of inpatient unit
5. Help family secure assistance of other home caregivers, if indicated
6. Prepare equipment/care proposal for submission to third-party payer, communicate with payer during approval process
7. Review planning checklist throughout the predischarge process and immediately prior to discharge

### Respiratory Therapist Responsibilities:

1. Investigate availability of home care vendors and services provided in child's area of residence
2. Compile list of respiratory home care equipment, review with pulmonologist
3. Submit equipment lists to home care vendors for bids
4. Review with family bids received, and make recommendation as to which bid to accept (after consultation with physicians)
5. Provide instruction in all home respiratory care equipment
6. Review the planning checklist throughout the predischarge process and immediately prior to discharge

### Social Worker Responsibilities:

1. Assess family/child to determine psychosocial suitability for home ventilation, give data and recommendation to pulmonologist prior to initial discussion with family
2. Provide ongoing assessment and support of child and family
3. Assess family financial status, especially of availability of payment for home ventilation expenses

### Primary Nurse Responsibilities:

1. With nurse specialist, meet with family to give overview of program and planning process
2. Coordinate teaching of tracheostomy care, gastrostomy tube care, feedings, medications, respiratory assessment to parents and other home caretakers
3. Communicate to remainder of staff regarding #2
4. Ensure that proper documentation of teaching of caregivers takes place
5. Meet with clinical nurse specialist, family, durable medical equipment vendor, and home nursing agency before discharge
6. Assist family in developing home schedule for equipment maintenance and child's daily care routine
7. Meet with clinical nurse specialist and home nursing agency to update on progress, changes, and problems
8. Develop care plan to be presented to all home care nurses and filed with agency
9. Assist clinical nurse specialist in developing training program and training schedule
10. Meet with home care team on first training day to present nursing care plan, etc.
11. Establish discharge supply list needed, establish communications with materials services, order supplies
12. Establish communication book to compile parent's questions

### Occupational, Physical, and Speech Therapists Responsibilities:

1. Develop home treatment plan
2. Communicate plan to parents and home care nurses during training program

## APPENDIX F

# Home Ventilator Program—Multidisciplinary Planning Checklist

Date/Initials

__________ 1. Pulmonologist meets with family for initial discussion/consideration of home ventilator program.

2. Team members notified and established as follows:
   - ______ primary physician
   - ______ nurse specialist
   - ______ respiratory therapist (continuing care specialist)
   - ______ social worker
   - ______ primary nurse
   - ______ occupational therapist
   - ______ physical therapist
   - ______ nutritionist
   - ______ speech therapist
   - ______
   - ______
   - ______

__________ 3. Nurse specialist and primary nurse meet with family to provide overview of program and planning process.

__________ 4. Multidisciplinary planning meeting scheduled by nurse specialist and held. Decisions made regarding ventilator, oxygen, hospital bed, wheelchair, nursing, monitor, trach, etc.

__________ 5. Primary nurse develops home care plan.

__________ 6. Primary nurse determines skills to be taught, obtains documentation sheets.

__________ 7. Nature of third-party payment determined by social worker.

__________ 8. Initial contact with third-party payer made by nurse specialist.

__________ 9. List of respiratory home care equipment compiled by respiratory therapist and reviewed by nurse specialist and primary physician.

__________ 10. Bid letters submitted to appropriate vendors by respiratory therapist.

__________ 11. Bids received and reviewed with family, vendor selected and notified, bid forwarded to nurse specialist.

__________ 12. Nurse specialist arranges meeting with vendor and family.

__________ 13. Family, assisted by primary nurse, clinical nurse specialist, and respiratory therapist, devises schedule for equipment maintenance at home.

__________ 14. Family makes decision about home nursing care, with consultation from nurse specialist and primary nurse.

__________ 15. Proposal submitted to third-party payer by nurse specialist.

__________ 16. Proposal accepted.

__________ 17. Nurse specialist and primary nurse plan home care teaching program for all caregivers.

__________ 18. Primary nurse, clinical nurse specialist, and parents meet with home care nursing agency.

__________ 19. Training schedule circulated to family and team members. Primary nurse assigns preceptors for all caregivers. Agenda for first day of training:

______ Nursing care plan presented

______ Introduction to family dynamics, program philosophy

______ Introduction to team members

______ Training schedule

__________ 20. Respiratory care equipment manuals provided to family.

__________ 21. Prior to discharge, all caretakers must demonstrate proficiency in the following skills (on each of three separate dates):

______ Cardiopulmonary resuscitation
______ All respiratory equipment
______ Trach care
______ Gastrostomy tube care or other feeding procedures
______ Respiratory assessment and intervention
______ Administration of all medications
______ Other specialized instruction

__________ 22. Primary nurse ensures that family has home care plan for occupational therapy, physical therapy, dietary, and speech therapy.

__________ 23. Nurse specialist coordinates and schedules first follow-up visit.

__________ 24. Primary nurse arranges meeting with nurse specialist, vendor, nursing agency, family, primary nurse, and respiratory therapist.

## Sample Interview Questions to be Used by Parents in Interviewing Home Care Nurses

What is your nursing background? Any pediatrics? Any ICU?
Where were you educated?
How are you qualified for *this* position?
What do you like, dislike about nursing?
What have been your rewards, disappointments in your career?
If this is an employment change: Why are you changing? *or* Why are you applying without experience?
Describe a crisis you handled well.
What nursing skills are you most proud of?
What do you think would be your biggest adjustment in coming to work with our child?
What about yourself would you like to improve or strengthen?
What patients give you the most satisfaction? Most frustration?
What do you expect as a typical shift in working in our home?
What activities outside nursing do you think have helped make you a better nurse?
Do you smoke? Do you like dogs, cats?

# Index